COMING BACK

Coming Back

A Guide to Recovering from Heart Attack

REVISED EDITION

KEITH COHN, M.D.
DARBY DUKE, R.N.

Illustrated by Craig Stilwell

Addison-Wesley Publishing Company, Inc.
READING, MASSACHUSETTS   MENLO PARK, CALIFORNIA
NEW YORK   DON MILLS, ONTARIO   WOKINGHAM, ENGLAND
AMSTERDAM   BONN   SYDNEY   SINGAPORE   TOKYO
MADRID   BOGOTÁ   SANTIAGO   SAN JUAN

Library of Congress Cataloging-in-Publication Data

Cohn, Keith, 1935.–
  Coming back.

  Bibliography: p.
  Includes index.
  1. Heart—Infarction—Patients—Rehabilitation.
2. Coronary heart disease—Patients—Rehabilitation.
3. Cardiacs—Rehabilitation. 4. Heart—Infarction—
Prevention. 5. Coronary heart disease—Prevention.
I. Duke, Darby, 1949–   . II. Title. [DNLM:
1. Coronary Disease—rehabilitation—popular works.
WG 113 C678c]
RC685.I6C63   1987   616.1'2306   86-28810
ISBN 0-201-05498-1

The authors and publishers have exerted every effort to insure that drug selection and dosage set forth in this text are in accord with current recommendations and practice at the time of publication. However, in view of ongoing research, changes in government regulations and the constant flow of information relating to drug therapy and drug reactions, the reader is urged to check the package insert for each drug for any change in indications of dosage and for added warnings and precautions. This is particularly important where the recommended agent is a new and/or infrequently employed drug.

Cover design by Frances Fleming
Text design by Dede Cummings
Set in 11-point Baskerville by Camden Type 'n Graphics, Camden, ME

ABCDEFGHI-DO-8987

First printing, April 1987

TO BUDDY LANGSTON,
our colleague and friend,
who cared and loved
and lived life abundantly

We are enormously grateful to Joseph Madrid for his invaluable help in preparing the first edition of this book.

KEITH COHN

DARBY M. DUKE

Contents

Foreword

ONE OF THE MOST difficult tasks for the physician is that of stating clearly and concisely to the heart patient in lay language just what is happening to him or her. Yet this task is important, since fear of the unknown—or rather fear of not knowing—is frequently more devastating to the patient than the medical setback itself is. *Coming Back* is a precise and comprehensible book that touches on all aspects of what the coronary patient wants and needs to know.

The authors nicely analyze the kinds of care, the hospital stay, the posthospital convalescence—including the all-important rehabilitation period—and even the seemingly complicated electronic equipment. In addition, because there has been so much emphasis on coronary bypass surgery, both in the lay press and in medical journals, the authors wisely stress the many other, nonsurgical approaches that offer comparable recovery results. Contrary to popular opinion, certainly not every patient with coronary artery disease is a candidate for surgery.

The dominant theme of this book is how to cope intelligently and effectively with a heart attack if it surfaces unexpectedly or prematurely. But there are lessons here as well for the reader who has not yet suffered a heart attack. If you live long enough, you will generally manifest some deterioration of your cardiovascular system. *Coming Back* shows you how to postpone or prevent that occurance as effectively as possible.

Norman E. Shumway, M.D.
Professor of Cardiovascular Surgery
Stanford University School of Medicine
Leading pioneer in cardiac transplantation

What This Book Is About

A HEART ATTACK is a frightening event that afflicts nearly one and a half million Americans every year. In addition, several million others develop some form of coronary disease. It's evident we face a problem of epidemic proportions.

But what is often overlooked is that a vast number of people who have suffered heart or coronary damage make a complete or nearly complete recovery and resume healthy, active, busy lives. Presidents Dwight D. Eisenhower and Lyndon B. Johnson, for instance, suffered heart attacks and still were able to continue their political careers. Many other famous figures in entertainment, business, the sciences, and the arts have also bounced back—some from bouts of coronary pain, others from full-fledged heart attacks.

Such people made their comebacks not only because of good medical care—monitoring, drug administration, and other therapy—but, most important, because they decided to take an active role in their care.

Coming Back describes the first part of the process, explaining what goes on in the hospital, what certain drugs do, and other hospital-related things. But we are mainly concerned with the second part—helping you get back on your feet once

1

you're back at home. It shows how you can overcome lingering fears and anxieties and help yourself back to a normal life or as nearly a normal life as circumstances permit.

And if you've been fortunate enough not to have any coronary problems in the first place, *Coming Back* shows you how they may be avoided.

The book has thus been written with the following points in mind:

- The information is presented from the *patient's viewpoint*, not the doctor's or nurse's. It is therefore expressed in layman's terms. At the same time, extensive additional information is offered in the back of the book which may be of interest to those who want to know more (see "Further Explorations").

- The information is presented like a *smorgasbord or salad bar*. You don't have to help yourself to everything. Feel free to skip the chapters that don't seem to apply to you. (If you don't smoke or drink, for example, or don't have chest pains or heart-rhythm disturbances, then you really don't care about them, and it's O.K. to skip those parts.)

- The information is presented in clear, *bite-sized, easily digestible* chunks. All chapters are short—usually only a few pages each.

- The information is presented in as *interesting and lively* a manner as is possible. Why should a helpful book be dull? We have tried to write this in a warm, personal, sympathetic, and above all interesting style. We have tried to encourage your involvement and awareness by providing self-diagnostic questionnaires, diagrams by which you can compare yourself to others, charts showing the odds for different kinds of health risks, and illustrations that clearly explain medical concepts and principles yet avoid a heavy medical and anatomical look unless absolutely required to make a point understandable.

- The information is *practical and current*. When we did not feel information was useful, we did not put it in. When it seemed to be a subject people were interested in (we get a lot of questions about coronary bypass and angioplasty, for instance—even from people who probably would not be candidates for the procedure), we gave it the space it deserved. The book is filled with useful tips to help you deal with threatening feelings and murky emotions, learn how to quit smoking, change your eating habits so meals become *more* rather than less interesting, and much more.

Although the book is intended for heart and coronary patients, many may want their families and friends to read it—if only to avoid what they themselves have suffered.

Ready to start your comeback? Turn the page.

1

Like a Bolt from the Blue:
Days 1–3

PERHAPS IT BEGAN as a burning, constricted feeling, a dull or heavy pain—the worst pain you have ever felt. Or perhaps it was simply a vague ache or discomfort, virtually unnoticed, even not noticed at all. Perhaps you thought you had indigestion, and even your doctor may have had difficulty telling that it was not simply an overdose of lasagna at dinner. Or perhaps you suddenly felt very weak, began sweating profusely, experienced a sense of impending doom, indeed, actually passed out.

There are many ways a heart attack can occur. It may have happened while you were sleeping, eating, driving, or at work. Like a bolt from the blue, it may have happened suddenly, without warning, at any time of day or night. On the other hand, it may have been preceded by hours, days, or even weeks of vague chest pains or general feelings of not-so-well-being. It may have been preceded by some exertion—gardening, lifting, playing tennis, even making love—or it may not. It may have been precipitated by emotional stress—conflict with your boss, an argument with another driver, great upset in the family—or it may not. Indeed, a heart attack is often preceded by *no* exertion or provocation whatsoever.

5

Doctors would prefer that there be as little time as possible between the onset of a heart attack and entry into the hospital, but it seldom happens that quickly. While people around you may have thought you looked ill—sweaty, pallid—you may have insisted you were O.K., maybe argued about what should be done, finally agreed to take an aspirin or Alka-Seltzer or lie down for a nap. Finally, someone called a doctor or the hospital and, perhaps after further debate about how to get you there (drive yourself? call an ambulance?), one way or another you wound up in the emergency room.

Then things probably began to happen very rapidly. The nurse or physician, suspecting a possible heart attack, ordered you onto a gurney or bed. Intravenous fluids were started in your arm. Blood samples were drawn. An electrocardiogram was taken. Wires were attached to your chest and connected to a monitoring device. Perhaps a chest x-ray was taken. Physicians and nurses probed with hands and listened with stethoscopes and asked a great many questions: How did you feel? What did you eat? Where, exactly, was the pain?

Then there came the decision whether or not to hospitalize you, and the physician confronted you and your family with the matter. Again, you may have protested that you were "basically O.K.," that you had a lot of things to do and had to get home, and you may have felt angry toward the hospital staff and your family for insisting that you were sick.

At about this point, however, you may also have begun to realize the enormity of the situation, a concern that became magnified when you began thinking back to the real world: Relatives would have to be called, the boss or subordinates notified, scheduled events cancelled. A thousand fears, worries, and questions may have surfaced. Will I be disabled, an invalid? Will I die? Will I be able to work, play, have sex, lead a normal life again? All the while, confusion reigned, because the amount of information being given you was either too little or so profuse that you would have had difficulty following it even if you weren't being given sedatives.

Finally, you were transferred to the coronary care unit (CCU) or similar intensive-care facility. There you were surrounded by an array of uncommon-looking, even frightening, electronic devices. Again, wires were placed on your chest and connected to a monitoring instrument at the central nursing station, where nurses continuously monitored your heart's electrical activity and heartbeat, as well as, perhaps, your blood pressure and respiration rate. You may have received oxygen through small nasal tubes. Periodically you were given intravenous solutions as well as medicines for everything from sleeping to heart-rhythm stabilization.

During this time you may actually have felt perfectly well. You had had your episode of chest pain and it disappeared and you just wanted to get out of there and go home. On the other hand, you may have experienced recurring bouts of chest pain, weakness, shortness of breath, or irregular heart rhythm. Thus, you may either have found yourself in a quiet room—waiting for something to happen, introspective, contemplative—or you may have found yourself critically ill, with a flurry of activity about you from time to time.

Of course your normal living habits were affected. Because of the diet prescribed by your physician, your meals—meager, semiliquid, salt-restricted—varied greatly from what you were used to. Depending on the severity of your heart attack, you may have found yourself restrained by your physician from doing your usual activities: not allowed to get out of bed, wash, shave, sit in a chair, even go to the bathroom (instead forced to use a bedside commode). Exercise, if any, probably consisted of a nurse or physical therapist helping you with simple arm and leg movements. These alterations in your normal activities you probably found demeaning and confusing, if not indeed frightening.

All of the above describe the first two or three days following a heart attack. If you are at this point, you and your family are confronted with one of the most important events in your lives, with many implications, both immediate and long-term. At the moment you may feel a tremendous sense of helplessness, like a *hostage* trapped in the coronary care unit, required to follow restrictions and instructions, some of them uncomfortable, some of which you may disagree with, many of which make little sense. Even if you have not been through such a traumatic experience—if, for instance, you are suffering from angina, the chest pains of coronary disease, or if you have had a bypass operation or angioplasty—

that can still be very unsettling, and you may have many worries and doubts about the future.

However, most heart patients eventually come through the hospitalization with little difficulty. Many make a comeback to a completely or nearly completely active, productive, exciting life—often more enjoyable than the one they had before.

And that's what this book is about: coming back.

2

In the Hospital: What's Going On Around Here?

IF YOU ARE STILL in the coronary care unit (CCU) or elsewhere in the hospital, this chapter may help you understand what's going on—who those people are that are checking your progress, what instruments they are working with, what the hospital routine is about. (If you have been discharged from the hospital, you may want to skip this chapter and move on to Chapter 3.)

Let's start with the people.

Medical Personnel

The attending physician may be your family doctor, an internist, or a cardiologist (or all three). His or her job is to act as the quarterback for the medical team, to diagnose and treat your condition and counsel you and your family.

The coronary care unit nurse, a nurse who specializes in the care of heart disease, constantly watches patients when they are first admitted to the hospital, monitors the vital signs, administers any medication or therapy prescribed by the physician, watches for adverse psychological reactions and

9

tries to help alleviate them, and in other ways is the heart patient's primary contact with all the medical specialists involved. You should consider the nurse, whether in the CCU or elsewhere, a valuable immediate and primary resource, both in the early, unsure beginning and later on, when you've returned home and may need to telephone for advice.

Other members of the recovery team are the physical therapist, dietician, occupational therapist, and psychological counselor or clergyman, although not all of these specialists are present in all hospitals.

The physical therapist is an expert in body movements and exercise, and will show you how to exercise for maximum benefit without straining the heart and blood vessels.

The dietician can explain what eating habits may have contributed to—and could aggravate further—the heart disease, and can develop menus of safe foods for you.

The occupational therapist can show you how to cope with activities after your release—how to bathe, cook, garden, and so on, in ways that pose the least stress for your heart and cardiovascular system.

A psychological counselor—psychologist, psychiatrist, minister, priest, rabbi—can help you cope with the fears, doubts, and anxieties that inevitably follow a heart attack. Don't hesitate to call on any of these people for advice.

In many hospitals the doctor and nurse will assist you in these various areas.

Equipment and Instruments

The coronary care unit (or similar intensive-care facility) is designed to allow maximum patient observation and care. However, the specialized electronic monitoring devices, which are usually located near your bed, can be intimidating indeed. The purpose of these devices is to relay moment-to-moment information about the electrical activity of your heart to the central nursing station, where it is under constant surveillance by the nursing staff. This information is available as it is happening, but the central nursing station equipment also has a memory capability, so that the staff can compare how your heart is operating now with how it was operating a few minutes ago.

Here are what the various instruments in the CCU do:

ELECTROCARDIOGRAM.   When your doctor wants to print out a complete record of your heart's electrical activity and rhythm, an electrocardiographic machine is often wheeled into your room. This records the heart's electrical activity on graph paper. The electrocardiograms (also called ECG or EKG) tell how fast the heart is beating and whether there are any irregularities in the heart rhythm. Electrocardiograms are taken when you are first admitted to the hospital and for two or more days afterwards, since changes in the electrical patterns help prove whether or not a heart attack did indeed take place.

It might be of interest for you to know that, even after the heart is completely healed from an attack, in the subsequent months or years to come, the ECG often continues to show a permanent sign, an imprint, of the previous heart attack, and this record can be used to help doctors keep an eye on your heart in the future.

THE OSCILLOSCOPE.   A slightly different kind of electrocardiogram can be used for continuous *monitoring* surveillance of the moment-to-moment changes in the rhythm of the heart. Small discs called electrodes are stuck to your chest and are attached by wires to devices called oscilloscopes, one of which is usually located in your room and another at the central nursing station. The oscilloscope is like the screen of a television set, only it shows wavelike lines, which represent the electricity of your heart. This electrical information is relayed to the central nursing station, where doctors and nurses can immediately see what is happening and be alerted to any unusual or unexpected changes in the behavior in the heart. This information may be processed by a computer that specially analyzes and files any changes in the rhythm.

TELEMETRY.   Some monitoring systems are not connected to the oscilloscopes by wires. Rather, electrodes attached to your chest relay ECG signals to the central nursing station via

Heart monitor

radio transmission. This telemetry is used not only in some coronary care units but also sometimes for patients moved to a less intensive care setting. Telemetry permits you to move about more freely, since you are not constrained by wires, and the medical staff can watch your reactions while you walk around the room or ward.

MONITORING OF PRESSURES WITHIN THE HEART. In most cases, your blood pressure is taken using the typical arm cuff and stethoscope. In some heart attacks, however, the blood pressure, and other pressures within the heart and lungs, can be watched by means of a small tube inserted into the arteries and veins. It is even possible to "float" a thin tube through the veins and heart into the lungs to record pressures there. Such devices are usually reserved for patients who require more intensive monitoring, and they may be helpful in deciding whether any change in therapy need be initiated.

TELEVISION MONITORS. In some hospitals, if you are in a room out of sight of the nursing staff, a TV camera transmits a closed-circuit picture to the central nursing station, so the nurses have a clear view of you at all times.

INTRAVENOUS FEEDING.   Most patients in the coronary care unit are given a small needle or tube in their vein so that the doctor or nurse may give medication at a moment's notice. In many cases, a glass bottle or plastic bag is attached to the needle with clear plastic tubing, so that you can be fed with sugar water or provided with a constant "drip" of medicines, if needed.

So much for instruments and equipment. What about the hospital regimen?

Hospital Activities

We will not get into medication and diet here; they are covered in later chapters. (Some of these medications are explained in Chapters 8 through 11 and also in Appendix A. Diet is described in Chapters 16 and 17 and Appendixes B through G.) However, we would like to talk a little about exercise. Surprised? Yes, it starts in the hospital.

In many places, you get exercise while you are still in bed in the CCU or intensive-care unit. A nurse or physical therapist may raise the head of your bed so that you are nearly sitting up, then move your hands up and down in circular motions in the air and flex your legs, wrists, and ankles. This activity is called *passive range-of-motion exercising,* because someone other than you is providing the energy for the movement. By the second or third day of your convalescence, perhaps, you'll be asked to perform these exercises by yourself *(active range-of-motion exercises).* At about this time also, you will be encouraged to wash your own face and hands and brush your teeth, and you will be allowed some TV watching and light reading.

After a while, you will be allowed to do the range-of-motion exercises sitting in a chair. You may feel faint at first, owing to a temporary drop in blood pressure caused by your going from complete bed rest to the more demanding activity

Passive
range-of-motion
exercise

Active
range-of-motion
exercise

in a chair. However, this will go away as you begin to move about and become more active. Of course, the degree of activity and length of time devoted to exercise will vary from patient to patient, depending on the severity of the heart attack.

After you have been transferred out of the CCU to a regular hospital room or ward, you will be asked to do your exercises in a standing position. Later, you will be asked to walk about in your room or the hospital halls, and you will probably be expected to count your own pulse carefully. At the same time, you will advance from taking sponge baths to taking tub baths or showers, using standard toilet facilities, and to playing cards or writing letters.

In the few days prior to your discharge from the hospital, the nurse or physical therapist may assist you in climbing stairs, beginning with three or four steps and progressing to short flights.

A Word About Doctor's Orders

We see two rather interesting phenomena among patients: Some make nervous wrecks of themselves and their families (and their physicians) by charging into their recovery and compulsively trying to follow everything the doctor says to the letter. Others simply ignore everything the doctor says and, for example, overexert themselves or fail to take their medications. Neither kind of behavior is desirable.

The thing to understand is the difference between orders and advice.

In general, *advice* is what your physician recommends about such things as diet and exercise. It is just that—advice—and that means modifications can be made. (Of course you don't have to stick to your diet during celebrations.)

Orders, on the other hand, apply to medications (and anything else the doctor particularly emphasizes). It is important not to miss medications, switch them around, change doses, or in other ways tamper with the program since otherwise they not only might not work but might actually be harmful.

End of speech.

The Future

While in the hospital you will probably be getting a lot of instructions and advice about medication, diet, and so on, which you are supposed to follow once you get home. The rest of this book is intended to assist in that, so that during the forthcoming weeks and months, you can get back to the best state of health possible.

However, simply having this book in your possession will do nothing for you. It must be read, perhaps more than once, until you know the information is working for you. *You and your participation* are the key to your recovery.

3

The Physician Within

WHY DON'T WE pause for just a moment and speak of something we consider to be very serious and important. You might even relax, close your eyes, and have someone read this chapter to you; let it soak in.

Let's face it, the role you play in getting well and staying well is essential. There is a powerful life force in each of us—a will to live, to survive, an energy that stands squarely against illness and infirmity. And, after all, who is better suited than you to join forces with that natural healing process taking place in your own body?

Yes, there's a struggle going on—a struggle to get well. And of course, during an illness you may find yourself feeling afraid, uncertain, a little sorry for yourself. But instead of being swallowed up by these emotions, these reactions that grab hold of you, you can put them in perspective: by realizing the importance of your own participation in this struggle to bring the healing, vital energies in touch with that part of your body which is in need of them.

First of all, you can begin by trying to understand a bit about the situation. Sometimes we are afraid because we don't know what's going on, what to expect. How does the

17

heart function? What goes wrong? "How can I be helped and how can I help myself?" So you need to delve into the secrets of the medical profession—hence, this book. By prying open this mysterious "black bag," you can begin to replace that nagging fear with some understanding. You need to recognize that you are not helpless, that, instead, you have an active part to play in your own recovery.

An illness, after all, is not purely physical; it involves all of you: your mind, body, instincts, and feelings. You are like a giant interconnected conglomerate—consisting of a think tank, business offices, chemical labs, refineries, mills, farms, cafeterias, a large diverse secretarial pool, even a tiny chapel. And if any part malfunctions, the organization may be threatened. Your mental and emotional outlook are every bit as critical to your health as are the organs and tissues themselves. So you need to begin to think and feel with a *new attitude,* one that comes from deep within your inner being— one that watches patiently and knows, and that can guide you back toward health.

Probably the last thing you want to hear is someone telling you, "don't worry, everything will be OK." Of course, a life crisis like this shakes you to your very roots. And certainly it is hard to see it as anything but a terrifying accident or a disaster. But as long as you are here, why not look at the possibilities, the opportunities? We have all heard stories about people who come through an illness and appear stronger than ever. "He's a changed man!" "She's a new woman!" In a crisis you are aroused to look seriously at yourself, at what your life is all about, at what is really important. You are jolted into a courageous inquiry into all those questions you have become so used to pushing aside, questions that help you rediscover yourself, your purpose, and your own strength.

So just for a moment, along with the uncertainty, fear, and impatience, you need to become quiet, to listen to the vibration of your body, and to feel the wonder and vitality of your being. Turn inward for a moment and search for that special sensitivity that encompasses everything: your illness, the healthy structures of your body, and the wisdom of nature. Let the healing energies circulate through your body; let them bathe all your tissues. You need to know, to feel with a certain intuitiveness that you can get well—or at the very least, feel better. We are not talking about false or impossible expectations, but about a realistic hope, one that brings purpose and confidence. You can begin to discover and to trust in the intelligence of your own body and the work of healing.

In the same way, you can begin searching for a more nourishing relationship with your doctors, nurses, other health professionals, and your loved ones—opening up to their compassion, judgement, and skilled craftsmanship, to that authentic part of every human being that has the force of healing within.

4

Feelings: Frustrations, Gripes, Tensions, Blues

JOHN ABBOTT, 55, a heavy-equipment operator, suffered a heart attack but recovered uneventfully. In the hospital his physician advised him to follow a low-cholesterol diet, to stop smoking, to avoid emotional stress, to eliminate heavy work temporarily, and to undertake a progressive physical exercise program. Shortly after his admission to the hospital, his chest pains disappeared and he had no additional symptoms. Thereupon he repeatedly demanded to be released, insisting that he hadn't had a heart attack but only some stomach disorder and heartburn. Four days after his discharge from the hospital, Abbott (not his real name) was discovered by his wife trying to move a heavy couch in the living room. He was also smoking a cigarette. A heated argument followed, and Abbott stomped angrily out of the house, leaving his wife confused and in tears.

Louis Meehan (also not his real name), 37, had only recently been promoted to vice-president in a metropolitan bank, when he suffered a heart attack accompanied by severe chest pain. He, too, recovered uneventfully, but weeks after his release from the hospital, when he should have been functioning almost normally, he continued to lack energy, was tired much of the time, felt low and discouraged, and had little motivation toward both his job and his previous interests. Formerly a talkative, outgoing person, he became quiet and withdrawn and oftentimes just sat around sadly and moped.

Until her heart attack, Eva Steinfield, 45, had been an active housewife, caring for three children as well as holding down a part-time job. Four months after leaving the hospital, however, she was unable to keep up with shopping and cleaning, had to beg out of her share of the car pool, and relied more and more on her husband to cope with the household and make decisions about the kids. Moreover, her life virtually centered around telephone calls and office visits to her physician, to whom she expressed concerns about a variety of aches and pains and repeatedly asked him about her medicines, potential remedies she had read about in magazines, and so on.

Are these patients acting ridiculously? Perhaps. But their responses are extremely common. Nearly everyone who has a heart attack appears to develop some emotional problem, and although changes in personality or manner may seem eccentric, they are not hard to understand, considering the stressful circumstances. Indeed, they can be viewed as being the *reasonable results* of one's having to face a life-threatening experience. Often some outside assistance—from a physician, nurse, psychologist, clergyman, or relative—is required to help with the adjustment.

The thing to understand is that millions of others who have had a heart attack have reacted in similar ways, but, generally speaking, with time and guidance, have outgrown these reactions.

In the CCU

If you were hospitalized for a heart attack in the coronary care unit (CCU), probably your first reaction was one of disbelief. Is this really happening to *me?* The shock of feeling fine one moment and finding yourself in a hospital bed the next, connected to heart telemetry and electrocardiogram wires, is overwhelming. It is an altogether unreal experience, especially if there was no warning. With some patients, this feeling is even expressed briefly as outrage at the fact that blind fate has singled them out for this personal tragedy, and they lash out at their families and the hospital staff.

In the next few hours or days, disbelief gave way to anxiety. You recalled friends and acquaintances who had had heart attacks. Had you considered them "washed up"? Did you wonder if you were washed up yourself? What about the job? Would there be money problems? Would your role in the family change? Would you be able to have sex again? What *does* the future hold?

Even if you were feeling O.K., you might have found yourself just waiting around for some disaster to happen—which, of course, simply added to the anxiety. Thus, you may have become intensely interested in your surroundings, closely observing every movement in the CCU, perhaps staring for hours at the screen of the telemetry unit monitoring your heart. Or you may have had difficulty concentrating, became easily distressed, and found it hard to remember or comprehend instructions (a good reason for hanging on to this book, so that you can review the things you were told and have forgotten). Many patients at this stage experience talkativeness—probably as a way of releasing nervous tension—as well as restlessness, sleeplessness, sweating, or trembling.

By the end of the first week in the hospital, you may have felt completely discouraged and depressed, worried about your future, perhaps even panicky.

If, as you read this, you are still in the hospital, you should try not to let these anxieties overwhelm you and create mischief later on. Talk over your feelings and fears with the hospital staff. That's what they're there for.

Coming Home

What is it like after you have been discharged from the hospital? At the very least you may be troubled by a number of minor complaints: strange aches and pains, sleeplessness, fatigue. These symptoms may seem to crop up all the time, and, of course, the more they occur the worse you feel, and you and your family may become convinced that a disaster lurks around every corner.

What is really happening, however, is that you've become emotionally *tied* to all of this. You have become more concerned with and introspective about yourself and your body, so that you notice every little ache and pain, even though your physician might already have judged them insignificant. As for the fatigue, you may have less zip merely because of inactivity, muscular tension, or because you've been drained by this emotional onslaught.

Most of these kinds of complaints will probably begin to disappear as time goes by. The best attitude to take is to understand that they do occur, discuss them with your physician so he or she can evaluate their significance, then deliberately put yourself in a positive "healing" frame of mind.

What about the *major* complaints, the larger emotions? How are you handling the fact that you had a heart attack? That depends on the kind of person you are, for, as we saw with the examples at the beginning of this chapter, people handle stress in different ways. Following the numbing shock that occurs during the first few days, the disbelief and anger, you probably reacted to the event in one of four ways:

- You continued to have strong feelings of *anxiety,* dwelling—perhaps obsessively—on the potential future danger of your illness.

- You may have become moderately to seriously *depressed,* as banker Louis Meehan did. Perhaps you became more quiet and withdrawn, your movements became slower and less bouncy, you lost some appetite, lost interest in your job or other major hobbies, or experienced vague feelings of fatigue, discouragement, sadness, or anxiety, even began weeping. Indeed, you may have become unwilling to venture far from home, becoming absorbed in your own despondency to the exclusion of all other interests.

- Like John Abbott, you may have actually *denied* you really had an illness—simply did not accept that such a fearful thing had happened, ignored pleas to give up smoking, lose weight, keep regular doctor's appointments. Indeed, some people, believing the heart attack beyond their control, respond by simply rejecting it, not acknowledging that anything serious has happened, contesting the diagnosis, minimizing the extent of the illness, and disregarding any restrictions.

- Like Mrs. Steinfield, you may have become exceedingly *dependent* on your physician, family, and friends. Some patients may even tend to revere the physician as a godlike figure and to become extraordinarily dependent on everyone for emotional sustenance and physical assistance.

Anxiety, depression, denial, despondency. Any one or a combination of these can occur. And they often develop in the first month or so after a heart attack.

Acceptance

In all the welter of conflicting emotions, *acceptance* may be the hardest, but it is the one that gives you the best chance of returning to a normal life. Acceptance is a letting go of all the emotional constraints, a simple acknowledgment of the situation as it is, so that you can more *freely* continue with your life.

When you return home from the hospital, you will be confined to some extent for at least 2 to 3 weeks. You may reexperience some of the feelings you had immediately after your heart attack, and you may thus find yourself irritated by the restrictions, the limited physical area, the sounds of children squabbling, the lack of things to do. You may find that an oversolicitous spouse can make the adjustment difficult. You may be worried about curtailments in your income. You may wonder if you can get back to a normal sex life. How do you handle all of these problems?

In dealing with your family and spouse, it is important that all of you recognize the apprehensions everyone has and that these anxieties be talked about openly. Good communications and free expression of real feelings will tend to lessen fears and prevent angry outbursts. Group sessions, in which several families share common experiences, may also represent a valuable way to uncover vexing problems. Ask your physician or nurse for recommendations.

Money worries can be a real cause of anxiety. The important thing to appreciate is that the faster you regain your health, the sooner you may be able to return to work. With your acceptance of your disability and your willingness to participate in your own recovery, this will happen sooner, not later.

Similarly with sex: Heart disease does not impair sexual function. Patients who have suffered heart attacks are just as capable of having healthy and satisfying sex lives as they were before. After all, it was the heart that was affected by your attack, not the rest of the body.

What if your physician says that your heart attack was a serious one, that there is a possibility that you may not reach full recovery? We don't want to raise false fears here, but some patients with extremely severe angina or very severe congestive heart failure are limited to various extents and cannot return to a normal life. There are varying degrees of incapacity and disability, which determine the extent to which one can return to work and to full-time recreational activities. But there is no sense sitting around worrying about these possibilities. You should simply decide you're going to try and do the best you can to return to as full and active a life as possible.

Keeping yourself occupied with a positive attitude goes a long way toward minimizing most of these problems. (Avoid repeated use of tranquilizers and too much booze—they're no way to cope over the long haul.) Remember: *the life expectancy of most people who survive a heart attack is better than most people think,* and most people who have had an attack go on to lead their lives as before.

The secret is in (1) acceptance and (2) an intention to come back.

For the Spouse, Family, and Friends

DURING THE 14 days her husband was in the hospital for a mild heart attack, Sylvia Adams (a pseudonym, as are the others in this chapter) camped out at his bedside and kept copious notes on everything the staff members said. Later, when he had returned home, she insisted he follow every aspect of his come-back program to the letter. She threw out every high-calorie, high-cholesterol food item in the house; stopped buying ice cream, Mr. Adams's favorite food; and harangued him when he ordered it in a restaurant.

She kept careful track of his medications (he took eight pills a day), following him around with a glass of water until he took each one. She timed his exercises with a stopwatch and even tried to take his pulse. Every Friday she insisted they participate in a group discussion with other heart-attack couples—basically a good idea, but the time conflicted with his weekly poker game.

In short, Mrs. Adams followed Mr. Adams's recovery program very well. Mr. Adams found her attentions a damned nuisance and resented being watched all the time.

What should be a physician's advice here? It should be to Mrs. Adams: "Relax. It is unnecessary to follow each instruction *precisely*. Being too caring or rigid can be annoying or even demeaning. The suggestions being made are simply prudent ones that should be followed the majority of the time."

In other words, although the doctor's instructions about *medications* should be followed exactly, the other advice— about diet, exercise, and the like—can be given greater latitude.

A second case: When his wife suffered a serious heart attack that hospitalized her for 6 weeks, Hugh Carlson, 55, was devastated. They had been married for 34 years and she had never been ill. She had stood with him through lean, rocky years and only recently had they finally had the time and money to enjoy themselves. When he came to see her in the hospital, he paced the floor and was unable to relax and visit. At home he didn't eat and sat for hours with the light off, doing nothing.

When Mrs. Carlson came home to a program of rest and slow recovery, he sat by her bed, holding her hand and fidgeting and talking very little. He showed little interest in his business and left all decisions to his son. He refused to discuss the future, even the next day's events. When the public-health nurse stopped by to check his wife's progress, he was staring out the window. Mrs. Carlson was in tears because she was unable to talk things over with him and felt she could not make any progress without his assistance and support.

What could the nurse have told him? It could be something like: "Look, you're in this together. Offer understanding, sympathy, emotional support; be a listening post; offer some physical assistance. Don't dump a lot of sadness on her. And if you can't shake off that despondency, you should probably seek professional advice."

A third case: Mr. and Mrs. James Newcomb had been married for 27 years, and in all that time he never discussed any health problems with her. When he suffered a moderately severe heart attack, he became angry when she suggested he seek medical assistance. Then, when he was finally hospitalized, he would not permit her to discuss anything with his doctor or nurse. She was not informed of any part of his come-back program, not even what medications he was taking. Because he had a number of heart irregularities and a very slow heart rate, a permanent pacemaker was implanted in him, and after one month he was sent home.

After a while he began having a recurrence of angina. His wife could tell by his facial expressions, nervousness, and general physical appearance that he was now having chest pains, but he denied it vigorously when she asked about it. Indeed, one night he awoke in great distress and asked his wife to get his nitroglycerin for him, but when she asked about it the next morning he laughed and said, "You must have been dreaming."

Mrs. Newcomb knows her husband is a very proud man who doesn't want to admit his weaknesses or burden her with his problems. However, she would like to be informed of his health status and take part in dealing with his problems and planning for further solution. The problem is she doesn't know exactly how to approach him about her wishes. What should we tell her? We'll try to answer this in a minute.

Working as Partners

As the three examples make clear, a heart attack affects not only the patient but his or her partner, as well as close family and friends. How should they handle the change in roles, the change in household and work patterns, the complex emotional reactions (both the patient's and their own)?

In general, we offer five pieces of advice:

- Have a positive attitude; you can share and transmit your own healing energies to your loved ones.

- Let the heart-attack patient know that *you* are important, too. How you and the patient interact has a significant effect on the quality of *both* your lives. It's not just a one-way street.

- Open communication is very important. You must have a free and honest relationship that encourages expression and venting of emotions, even adverse feelings. Listen to what the other is saying. Try to understand what is being said from the other person's point of view as well as your own. Avoid constant argument, tension, hostility (read

Chapter 4 about the patient's feelings). Emphasize the positive while still being aware of any negative feelings.

- Be aware of whatever the plan is for recovery or plans for the future. These plans should be realistic and something that you can work on together. Be available to give assistance when needed and supportive of the things that you cannot help with.

- Seek guidance, if necessary. Certainly the Adamses, Carlsons, and Newcombs could have benefited with professional help in dealing with their relationships. It is best if both partners or parties agree to this, of course, but by all means get help for yourself if you feel you need it—that would be the kind of advice we would give Mrs. Newcomb, since she was unable to communicate with her balky husband. Discuss any difficulties with the patient's physician, if he or she is someone you can talk with, or the nurse in the coronary care unit or regular ward, or a marriage counselor or a clergyman. In this connection, you may find so-called "heart clubs" of value.

Facing the Future

Mrs. Ellis, 65, suffered a large heart attack shortly after she and her husband returned from a cross-country trip, and her doctor advised them to cancel their long-planned trip to Europe to visit a daughter and son-in-law. Mr. Ellis had recently retired and was enjoying his free time, and both had been looking forward to doing a good deal more traveling than they had been able to do in the past. The heart attack was, of course, a shock and tremendous disappointment to both of them, and they realized many of their plans would have to change. However, because they cared about each other and were open with each other, they were able to discuss their feelings and make realistic yet satisfactory plans for the future, postponing the trip for a few months.

In short, we cannot emphasize enough to spouses, family, and friends the importance of loving concern, open communication, realistic planning for the future, and lending your own strength.

6

How the Heart Works:
A Crash Course

WELL, BACK TO SCHOOL for a moment. In order to understand your particular heart condition and what you can do
about it, it is necessary to have an idea about what the heart
looks like and how it works. Briefly defined, the heart is a
pump—a hollow, muscular organ located slightly to the left of
center in your chest—which pumps blood through a series of
tubes, blood vessels, to provide oxygen and nourishment to
the tissues in the body.

How the Heart Is Built

As the illustration on the next page shows, the heart is divided into two sides, left and right, Each side has a lower
chamber called a *ventricle,* which pumps the blood out of the
heart, and an upper chamber called an *atrium,* which receives
the blood returned to the heart.

The walls of the heart are made up of muscle called the
myocardium, but this muscle is not the same thickness everywhere. The myocardium of the upper chambers (atria)
is quite thin compared with the myocardium of the lower

31

Exterior view

Aorta

Left atrium

Right atrium

Left ventricle

Right ventricle

Interior view

Aorta

Left atrium

Aortic valve

Mitral valve

Right atrium

Tricuspid valve

Left ventricle

Right ventricle

chambers (ventricles). The muscular wall of the left ventricle is three times thicker than that of the right. This powerful left ventricular muscle is often referred to as the "main pump" because, like milking a cow's udder, it squeezes the blood out of the heart to *all* parts of the body with every heartbeat. The heart fills with blood when it is resting (in *diastole*) and pumps the blood out during the contraction (in *systole*).

The upper and lower chambers of the heart are separated by two valves, called *atrioventricular* (AV) *valves.* The left one is called the *mitral* valve, the right, the *tricuspid.* These valves prevent blood from flowing back into the atria from the ventricles when the heart is beating.

Two other valves, called *semilunar valves,* separate the ventricles from the blood vessels that lead from the heart to the lungs and the rest of the body. The left valve is called the *aortic,* and the right valve is called the *pulmonary.* Their function is to prevent the return of blood from the aorta or the pulmonary artery to the ventricles when the heart is resting between beats.

Diastole   Systole

The closing of these valves as the heart beats—first the AV valves, then the semilunar—produces the "lub-dub" sounds a doctor hears when listening through a stethoscope placed on your chest. If the valves are faulty and do not close properly, he or she may hear a "murmur" as the blood leaks backward through these valves.

Go with the Flow

As the illustration opposite shows, the right side of the heart receives blood from all parts of the body. Blood is bright red when it is full of oxygen, but after it returns from the body to the heart, having nourished the tissues and given up a portion of its oxygen, the blood looks slightly bluish or purplish. This incoming blood flows into the right atrium (1 in the drawing), then through the tricuspid valve (2) and into the right ventricle (3), which, on the next contraction or heartbeat, squeezes the blood through the semilunar pulmonary valve (4) through the pulmonary artery (5) into the lungs, which replenish the blood with oxygen.

This oxygen-rich red blood then flows back through the pulmonary veins (6) into the left atrium (7) and through the mitral valve (8) into the left ventricle (9). At the next heartbeat, this left ventricle forcibly contracts its muscular walls and pushes the blood through the aortic valve (10) and out through the aorta (11) to the rest of the body.

How does the blood manage to get to and nourish the tissues? As the illustration shows, the oxygen-rich blood leaves the heart and travels to the tissues of the body through a system of blood vessels, hollow tubes called *arteries*. The aorta is the largest artery, and it divides into smaller arteries, which themselves divide into even smaller arteries—a system much like the limbs, branches, and twigs of a tree.

The smallest arteries empty into one end of a profuse network of tiny blood vessels called *capillaries*, which deliver to the tissues the oxygen and other nutritional substances that the body uses for fuel and energy. These capillaries supply the head, arms, legs and various organs in the abdomen, such as the liver and stomach—and, of course, the heart (the heart in effect feeds itself).

To head and arms

Right lung

Left lung

Aorta

11

Right lung 5

6

7

1 10 8

4

2 9

3

To abdomen and legs

Venous system

Arterial system

Capillary system

The circulatory system

The other end of the capillary network joins with the *veins*, which carry the oxygen-depleted blood back to the heart. The veins are initially small and become larger and larger until they all unite into the largest veins, called the *vena cavae*, which empty into the right atrium of the heart. This brings us full circle.

The heart, arteries, veins, and capillaries are collectively termed the *cardiovascular system*. This amazing circuit assures the adequate delivery of nutritional substances to all the body tissues.

The Heart's Own Arteries

The heart has its own system of arteries called *coronary arteries*, which serve to nourish the heart muscle (myocardium), so that the heart can continue to function as a non-stop pump. The coronary arteries are the fuel lines to the heart. They branch off the aorta, as the third illustration shows, cross over the outside of the heart wall, and penetrate the muscle itself, dividing repeatedly into smaller and smaller branches. The left main coronary artery divides into the left anterior descending artery, which supplies the front, and the circumflex, which goes to the left side and around the back of the heart. The right coronary artery curls around the right side and back of the heart, bringing blood to those regions.

The Beat Goes On

The heart beats about 100,000 times a day, with only a fraction of a second rest between beats. Most adults experience about 60 to 100 contractions a minute.

What causes these contractions is the heart's electrical system, which produces the normal rhythmic beating? A small group of cells, called the *sinus node* and located in the right atrium, send electrical impulses across the heart muscle, stimulating the muscles of the atrium and then those of the ventricle. When so stimulated, the muscle walls contract,

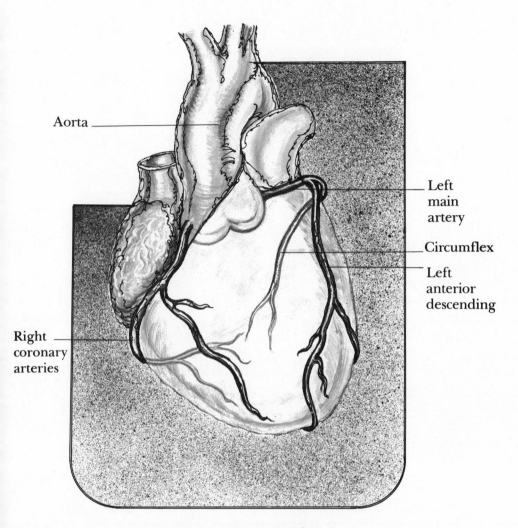

Aorta

Left main artery

Circumflex

Left anterior descending

Right coronary arteries

The coronary arteries

pumping the blood throughout the cardiovascular system. With it all, the heart pumps over 4,000 gallons of blood through the body each day.

Now, let us see how this crash course on the heart can help you understand your own heart or coronary disorder.

Clogged Pipes: Atherosclerosis and Coronary Disease

HOW DID YOUR HEART and blood vessels get to the state that they are in today? In all likelihood, it started when you were much younger, perhaps even in childhood. A narrowing or blocking of certain arteries began developing, caused by a condition known as *atherosclerosis,* commonly referred to as "hardening of the arteries" or "arteriosclerosis."

Atherosclerosis consists of fatty substances and other particles within the bloodstream collecting on the normally smooth inside walls of the arteries. The precise cause of this condition is not always known, but it may partly be due to or become worse as the result of smoking, high blood pressure, or excessive amounts of cholesterol and saturated fats in your diet.

Initially, atherosclerosis starts as a thin streak or plaque inside the wall of the artery, and as it grows, it begins attracting more and more cholesterol and fatty substances around it.

As these fatty substances accumulate, usually over a period of many years, the build-up becomes progressively thicker, and the channel inside the artery becomes steadily narrowed (see illustration on next page). In addition, the blood may stick to these fatty substances and clot, causing further clogging of the channel. (This blood clot is called a *thrombus.*)

Progressive obstruction of artery from atherosclerosis

The result of this narrowing is, of course, an interference in the flow of blood, which means certain tissues in your body aren't getting enough oxygen and other nutrients.

Effects of Atherosclerosis on the Heart

When an accumulation of these fatty substances or blood clots stop or severely restrict the flow of blood through the coronary arteries (the arteries of the heart itself), there may be two principal effects:

- *Angina pectoris:* There may be a *temporary* inadequacy in the supply of blood needed to meet the requirements of the heart tissue. This situation can cause feelings of pain or discomfort in the chest, called *angina pectoris* or simply "angina." The symptoms are transient, and no permanent changes nor damage to the heart muscle occurs.

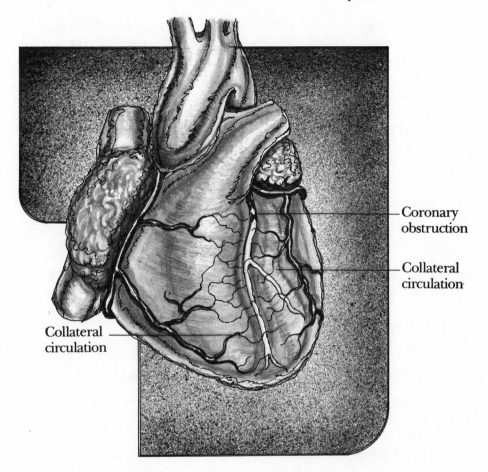

Coronary
obstruction

Collateral
circulation

Collateral
circulation

- *Myocardial infarction:* Otherwise known as a "heart attack,"
  "coronary," or "coronary thrombosis," this occurs when the
  blood supply becomes so restricted that it actually causes
  injury to the heart muscle.

It is possible to have coronary artery disease and *not* experience angina or a heart attack, either because the narrowing
of the arteries is not severe enough to interfere with the
nutrition of the heart or because there are enough other
arteries in the heart so that, when one is blocked, the blood is
routed to the same area through another, nearby artery. If

one coronary artery fails, a nearby one may establish new branches to service the deprived area of the heart. This development of cross-connecting branches is termed *collateral circulation*—see the illustration on the next page.

Angina pectoris, myocardial infarction, and other consequences of coronary disease, such as rate and rhythm disturbances and congestive failure, are described in greater detail in the next four chapters.

Other Problems Caused by Atherosclerosis

Atherosclerosis may also cause:

- *Stroke*—blockage in an artery supplying the brain, resulting in temporary or permanent damage and manifesting itself as some form of sudden paralysis or defect in speech or vision.

- *Blockage of the kidney artery*—causing kidney failure or high blood pressure.

- *Blockage in arteries to the legs*—causing pain in the calf, thigh or buttock, especially when walking.

Serious as atherosclerosis can be, your physician is more than familiar with how it's best handled. Between the two of you and the therapy we plan to lay out in this book, there is a reasonable chance it can be stabilized.

8

Chest Distress:
Angina Pectoris

WHEN YOU RUN for a bus or get into an argument, you're probably aware (at least afterwards) of your heart working especially hard: the heart demands more energy-producing fuel (oxygen and other nutrients) as it beats more vigorously and rapidly. Conversely, when you are sleeping or relaxed, the heart doesn't need to work particularly hard and it requires much less in the way of fuel.

When no coronary disease is present, the coronary arteries are able to supply an amount of blood to the heart muscle appropriate to its need. However, when coronary disease is present, the blood flow to the heart muscle is potentially restricted, and the more severe the coronary narrowing, the more limited the fuel supply to the heart. Although adequate amounts of blood may reach the heart muscle when you're relatively inactive, under circumstances of activity or anxiety a condition termed *coronary insufficiency* may develop. As the heart pumps more vigorously, not enough blood is able to reach the heart muscle because of the narrowed arteries. This may produce the chest pain, *angina pectoris*.

Physical
activity

Emotional
tension

Cold
weather

Heavy
meals

Conditions triggering episodes of angina

Symptoms

You may recall from the previous chapter that angina occurs when there is a "temporary" inadequate delivery of blood to the heart. That's why angina discomfort usually lasts only a few minutes or less and goes away if you rest or take medication.

The symptoms of angina vary considerably, and may be felt as a mild, vague feeling by some people and as a severe pain by others. Among the most commonly reported symptoms are a dull, pressing, weightlike, burning, or constricting sensation in the midchest or solar plexus. The pain may remain in the center of the chest or it may spread to the neck, lower jaw, shoulders, or down into either arm (more commonly the left arm) toward the elbow. It's a little different in everyone. And some folks feel nothing whatsoever even though there may be a transient inadequacy in blood supply to their heart.

The possible situations that can bring on angina are limitless. Some people have pain just walking around the block, while others, only after two sets of singles tennis. Some get angina when they have sex; others after a shouting match with their teenager. So that angina is often provoked by:

- Exertion

- Emotional stress

- Activity following a heavy meal

- Activity in cold, hot, or humid weather

- Sexual relations

Don't Be Fooled

Not every chest pain or ache is due to coronary disease or angina pectoris. Other conditions which are *not serious* often occur that may produce similar symptoms, which can be

frightening and may make you think you are having angina
or a heart attack. For example:

* Muscular spasms in the chest wall, often sharp or stabbing
  pains in a small area on one side of the chest.

* Diseases of the stomach or other parts of the gastrointestinal tract, including acid indigestion, ulcers, gallblad-
  der disease.

* Abnormalities of the spine.

* Pericarditis and pleurisy—inflammation of the sac surrounding the heart or lungs.

* Simple worry or anxiety.

When in doubt, check with your physician for proper diagnosis. No need to fret needlessly.

Another point: Though angina is due to atherosclerosis
most of the time, rarely we find no plaque blocking the
artery; instead spasm of the artery, a temporary constriction,
produces chest pain. This is sometimes termed "variant
angina."

Changes in the Frequency
and Severity of Angina

Many patients have angina lasting for years, yet they are only
minimally limited and never suffer a heart attack. Indeed, the
angina may even disappear. However, sometimes it may become more severe, and, if precipitously worse, may precede
a heart attack. And sometimes it may occur during hospitalization for a heart attack or appear after a patient is released
from the hospital following an attack.

Angina can be a possible *warning* of a more urgent condition, if the following occur:

* It becomes more severe over a period of time or develops
  with increasing frequency.

- It occurs as the result of progressively less activity or exertion.

- It persists after you have been discharged from the hospital following a heart attack.

- It begins to develop at night, waking you from a sound sleep.

- It persists for more than 10 to 15 minutes.

- The pain is severe enough to cause unusual perspiration.

- It is not readily relieved by rest or by taking more than three nitroglycerin tablets or the usually prescribed amount of nitroglycerin.

None of these signs is an absolute indicator of an impending problem, but you should check with your physician to be sure. If the discomfort is reasonably severe or unusual, have someone drive you to a nearby hospital emergency room. Your doctor or the staff on duty there can evaluate the situation and decide if there is cause for concern.

Diagnosis

The most helpful information for making the diagnosis comes from you. Your description of the symptoms you're feeling gives your physician a good idea of whether you have angina or not. He or she may then want to get an electrocardiogram or exercise test (also known as a stress test). And if these turn out to be suspicious, he or she may decide to gather more detailed information about your heart and recommend a coronary angiogram. We'll tell you about these tests later.

Treatment

Among the drugs commonly used to treat angina pectoris are nitroglycerin, some long-acting nitroglycerinlike drugs called *nitrates, beta blockers,* and some newer drugs called *calcium channel blockers.* Their objective is to reduce the demand by the heart for oxygen and other nutrients.

The nitrates are a group of drugs that help drop the blood pressure and reduce the amount of blood the heart has to pump, thereby decreasing the amount of oxygen required to nourish the heart muscle; angina pain thus disappears. Nitroglycerin, a short-acting nitrate, is taken under the tongue *during* an angina attack to speed the disappearance of the pain. Don't be worried about taking nitroglycerin; it's not dangerous (it's not the explosive kind) or habit forming and won't lose its strength with repeated use. The long-acting nitrates are taken at regular intervals, not during the pain but to *prevent* its recurrence. The many kinds of nitrates are explained in Appendix A.

Beta-blocking drugs slow the heart rate and diminish the vigor of the heart muscle contraction, thereby decreasing its workload and consequent demand for a large blood and oxygen supply, so that the angina is decreased or disappears. Calcium blockers lighten the workload of the heart, may slow it down, and relieve coronary artery spasm.

Watching Your Physical Activity

Pay attention to which activities bring on angina and try to avoid these. But in general, we do encourage physical activity. So walk as much as you can; you may even decide to join an exercise program. Be careful in extremes of weather. If you develop pain when exercising, stop what you are doing and rest, or sit down and take a nitroglycerin.

Another approach designed to lessen the likelihood of further narrowing of the coronary arteries is to eliminate principal risk factors by controlling high blood pressure, stopping smoking, dealing with emotional stress, beginning an exercise program, and eating right, a low-cholesterol or, if necessary, a weight-reducing diet. These are described later. Sometimes balloon angioplasty or coronary bypass surgery is required for stubborn angina cases; this is discussed in Chapter 25.

The Future

Angina pectoris may be uncomfortable or quite disabling, but, remember, it is eminently subject to successful therapy. Your symptoms can be effectively treated in most cases, the dangers may be minimized, and steps can be taken to prevent the problem from progressing.

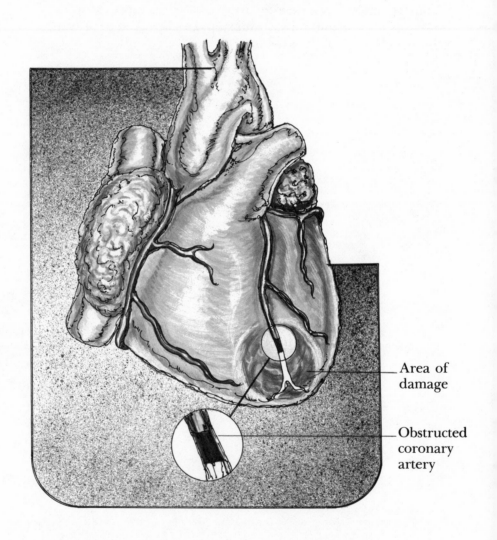

Area of
damage

Obstructed
coronary
artery

9

Heart Attack: The M.I.

THE CLASSIC PICTURE most people have of someone with a heart attack is of that person in an agony of pain ("the worst pain I've ever felt," some have described it), and indeed this may be the case. Yet, surprisingly, often there may be very little pain or discomfort during a heart attack.

What is a heart attack exactly? It happens when a coronary artery has become severely narrowed by atherosclerosis and also, possibly, when a small clot of blood settles on top of the fatty substance on the walls of the artery, clogging up the works and preventing blood from reaching the heart muscle. When the attack occurs, this area of the heart muscle becomes damaged because of the lack of blood supply. This heart attack is called a "myocardial infarction," "M.I.," "coronary," or "coronary thrombosis."

Symptoms

As we indicated in Chapter 1, a heart attack may become apparent to you in a variety of ways:

- It may cause pain in the chest or just below the rib cage in the solar plexus, occasionally spreading to one or both shoulders or upper arms, and may last for minutes or even hours. As mentioned, the discomfort may be rather mild, perhaps totally unnoticed, or it may be severe and may be accompanied by sweating, nausea, vomiting, weakness, or fainting.

- It may cause disturbances of the *rhythm of the heart* (see Chapter 10), either inconsequential or serious enough to require therapy—so serious they may occasionally lead to the heart's stopping. If this didn't happen within the first few hours, chances are it won't.

- It may cause interference with the pumping action of the heart, resulting in symptoms of *congestive heart failure* (see Chapter 11) or in a fall in blood pressure.

Prompt Attention

If you suspect you're having a heart attack, don't delay. Immediately call your doctor or go to a nearby emergency room. No harm is done if it turns out to be a false alarm.

Many people die needlessly from heart attack, because they do not get help quickly enough. The first few hours of an M.I. are the most crucial. Prompt care in a hospital with trained personnel can and does save lives. It's a good idea to be familiar with the resources for emergency help in your community. Many areas of the country have an all-purpose phone number—911; remember it. And it makes sense for family members to know cardiopulmonary resuscitation (CPR). You never know when an emergency is just around the corner.

The Rx Plan

Here's a brief summary of how your care might be approached:

* Monitoring in the CCU

* Rest

* Medications (A number of medications are commonly used to treat myocardial infarctions, some administered in pill form, some by injections, and some by intravenous infusions. Medications are utilized to strengthen the heartbeat, modify the blood pressure, control rhythm disturbances, and to make you more pain free and allow you to sleep. You can look up some of the drugs you might be taking in Appendix A.)

* Opening up, or bypassing, the obstruction. Necessary only in some cases; we'll talk more about this later.

* Beginning a cardiac rehabilitation program. And that's what the majority of the rest of this book is about.

Cooling It for a While

During the first few days (and especially the first few hours) following a myocardial infarction, the damaged heart is particularly sensitive, and any undue activity may bring about more chest pain, change in blood pressure, or heart-rhythm irregularity. Thus, complete bed rest is usually necessary for two or three days. During this time, and in the weeks to follow, the heart's own reparative processes begin to work, eventually forming a scar and strengthening the damaged tissue.

Doctors don't prescribe bed rest or limited activity without reason. Just as putting a broken arm in a cast allows the bone to rest and repair itself, reducing your physical activity and, thus, the work that the heart has to do, gives the injured tissue a greater opportunity for recovery. It simply takes time for your heart to heal.

The Future

Heart attacks vary greatly in the amount of damage done. Some myocardial infarctions are quite small and produce few long-term consequences—after recovery you can essentially return to a normal way of living. Other attacks are somewhat larger, and you may be obliged to modify your working and living habits to some degree in the months to come. In some cases the heart attack is so severe—with persisting congestive heart failure, angina, or rhythm disturbances (see the individual chapters on these subjects)—that substantial modifications must be made in activities and occupation. The point to remember, though, is that an enormous number of people who have had a heart attack return to an active and productive way of life.

The heart generally completes its reparative processes in two or three months. As we will show, this is not just time on your hands. There are a number of important programs to undertake to help you in your comeback.

10

Out of Sync: Rate and Rhythm Disturbances

IF YOU'VE EVER HAD too many cups of coffee or cigarettes or drinks, you may have noticed your heart seemed to "skip a beat"—that is, experience premature or early heart beats (called *extrasystoles*). Sometimes such skipped beats seem to happen for no particular reason at all, but in any case they are not an unusual occurrence, even in people with normal hearts, and are no cause for alarm.

The heart has its own electrical system, which produces an evenly timed, regular, clocklike beat. When relaxed, most adults have a heart rate between 60 and 80 beats per minute—slower if they are in good physical shape. Of course the heart beats faster (100–150 or more) during strenuous activity or emotional stress and slower during sleep or relaxation.

Rhythm Disturbances Due to Heart Attack

A heart-attack patient, however, may experience one of several rate and rhythm disturbances, which, if untreated, could become dangerous:

- Irregular heart rhythms: including increasingly frequent premature beats (also termed ectopic beats or extrasystoles) and atrial fibrillation (a totally irregular beat).

- Slower than normal heart rate (bradycardia).

- Faster than normal heart rate (tachycardia).

Let us consider these.

Irregular Beating of the Heart (Extrasystoles and Fibrillation)

Sometimes a heart attack can cause an irregularity in the heart's rhythm. Premature, or early, heartbeats (extrasystoles) can occur infrequently–that is, less than a few times a minute—or may appear with increasing frequency—more than 10 or 20 times per minute. Premature beats may actually lead to a very fast heart rate, a tachycardia. In atrial fibrillation, the rhythm of the heart is totally irregular and at times the heart beats excessively rapidly.

TREATMENT.   In the CCU, rare premature beats may require no therapy, whereas more frequent ones are treated with rhythm-suppressing drugs, such as lidocaine (Xylocaine) or procainamide. These are drugs administered intravenously which suppress premature contractions and prevent the appearance of a tachycardia. In some coronary care units, lidocaine is given even if no premature beats are seen, to *prevent* the emergence of potentially serious rhythm disturbances.

When premature beats occur after the first several days of the heart attack, they may be treated by drugs in pill form, such as beta blockers, quinidine, or procainamide, and many newer ones which can suppress or correct irregular heart rhythm. Atrial fibrillation is treated with either a digitalis preparation, a beta or a calcium blocker to slow the heart rate, or with one of the antiarrhythmic drugs to abolish this irregularity of rhythm.

Rapid Heartbeat (Tachycardia)

As indicated earlier, the heart rate will normally increase during physical activity or emotion, in order to supply more blood to the body tissues. There are times, however, when, unrelated to these normal conditions, the heart may spontaneously begin to beat excessively rapidly—a condition termed tachycardia. In many cases, this situation is of little or no concern and may quickly correct itself. In other cases, it may lead to there being a shortage of blood delivered to the tissues and a fall of blood pressure.

Among the symptoms of tachycardia are palpitations, a sense that the heart is racing, skipping, or beating irregularly; the feeling of faintness, weakness, confusion, or upset

stomach, owing to reduced blood supply to the tissues; shortness of breath, because of the backing up of blood in the
lungs; or chest pain, if an inadequate amount of blood is
reaching the heart muscle.

TREATMENT. The same medications used to treat irregular
heart rhythms are used to treat the tachycardias. In addition, in certain cases of tachycardia and atrial fibrillation, it
may be necessary to apply an electrical shock to the patient's
chest (often called *cardioversion*) in order to cause the heart
to resume its normal pace. A total discoordination of the
electrical activity of the heart is called *ventricular fibrillation*
and this requires immediate electric shock.

Slow Heartbeat (Bradycardia)

When the heart slows down to rates below 45 to 50 beats per
minute, it may (like tachycardia) lead to a deficiency of
blood reaching the tissues. The blood pressure may fall, and
one may feel dizziness, faintness, or confusion, or may even
pass out for a moment. Symptoms similar to those seen in
tachycardia may also appear. One cause of a very slow heart
rate is termed *heart block,* where an interruption of the electrical transmission in the heart takes place.

TREATMENT. As is true of irregular rhythms and tachycardia, slowing of the heart may require no therapy at all. In
rare instances, a drug such as atropine or isoproterenol
(Isuprel) may be injected in order to speed the heart.

In addition, when a patient has a very slow heart that does
not respond to drug therapy, an electrical *pacemaker* may be
used to speed the electrical impulses to the heart and cause
it to contract at a normal rate (see illustration on the next
page). This is a compact battery system, designed to deliver
a series of small electrical impulses to the heart muscle, usually at the rate of 60 to 75 times a minute. The pacemaker is
connected to the heart with an insulated wire which passes
through a vein to lie against the inner surface of the heart.

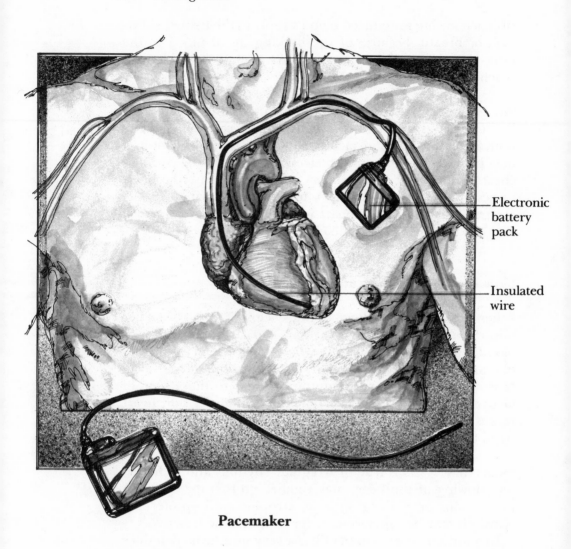

Pacemaker

Each electrical impulse from the pacemaker causes the heart to contract or beat. Some of the new pacemakers (called *A-V sequential* or *DDD*) are so sophisticated that they are able to coordinate the beating of the upper and lower chambers of the heart.

The Future

The disturbed heart rhythms, such as premature beats, atrial fibrillation, tachycardia, and bradycardia, may cause problems when they occur during or after a heart attack. Fortunately, the development of efficient cardiac monitoring equipment for the coronary care unit in the hospital to detect these abnormal rhythms has made early discovery and treatment possible and has resulted in a dramatic decrease in the number of fatalities from heart attacks among hospitalized patients.

Moreover, the physicians and nurses in the coronary care unit are trained specifically to recognize and treat rate and rhythm disturbances that may occur following a heart attack. There is always someone watching the heart monitors and ready to deal with any emergency. Today, CCU patients seldom have rhythm disturbances that cannot be readily corrected.

11

Problems Down at the Pump: Congestive Heart Failure

THE TERM "heart failure" is an unfortunate one—as well as misleading and frightening—since it certainly should not imply the heart has stopped or is in danger of stopping. However, *congestive heart failure* is the name given to the condition in which, when the heart muscle is weakened and its ability to pump impaired, blood backs up into the tissues and there is an inadequate supply of blood and nutrients delivered to the rest of the body.

This heart failure may be caused by a heart attack (from the damaged heart muscle), persistent high blood pressure (owing to the long-time pressure load under which the heart has been forced to labor), or a variety of other disorders, including valve defects, birth defects of the heart, and other diseases not discussed here. Whatever the cause, the effect is that the normal ability of the heart to pump blood declines, and the body begins to retain excessive quantities of salt and water.

Symptoms

Congestive heart failure may become apparent in the following ways:

- Fluids collect in the lungs and limbs.

- As these fluids accumulate, the lungs become congested, and shortness of breath results. This difficulty in breathing most commonly occurs after some physical activity, although it can also develop when you are lying down and be so severe that it may awaken you from a sound sleep, and you may find it necessary to prop yourself up in bed.

- Because fluids begin to seep through the thin walls of the capillaries and accumulate in the tissues, a swelling called *edema* develops in the ankles, legs, and sometimes even the abdomen. Edema is frequently first noticed as a tightness of shoes or clothing.

Treatment

Besides restricting your salt intake, your physician may prescribe the following medications:

- Different forms of digitalis, including digoxin and digitoxin—drugs that increase the pumping action (strength of contraction) of the heart.

- Diuretics or water pills—of which many types are available. These act to remove excessive amounts of salt and water from the body by causing increases in the amount of urination.

- Drugs that reduce the load on the heart. By relaxing the walls of the blood vessels and lowering the pressure against which the heart must pump, these medicines allow the heart to contract more effectively. It's as if you were carrying two suitcases up a hill and someone came along and lightened your load by carrying one of them.

The Future

Many patients feel tired or short of breath following a heart attack, not because of the heart's failure to pump effectively, but because they are out of condition—they have lost their normal body tone as the result of days and weeks of inactivity. There may also be anxiety arising from the stresses of the attack, and this, too, will cause fatigue.

If you are troubled with either of these symptoms, check it out with a physician. The danger is often not nearly as severe as it sounds, and appropriate therapy is generally available.

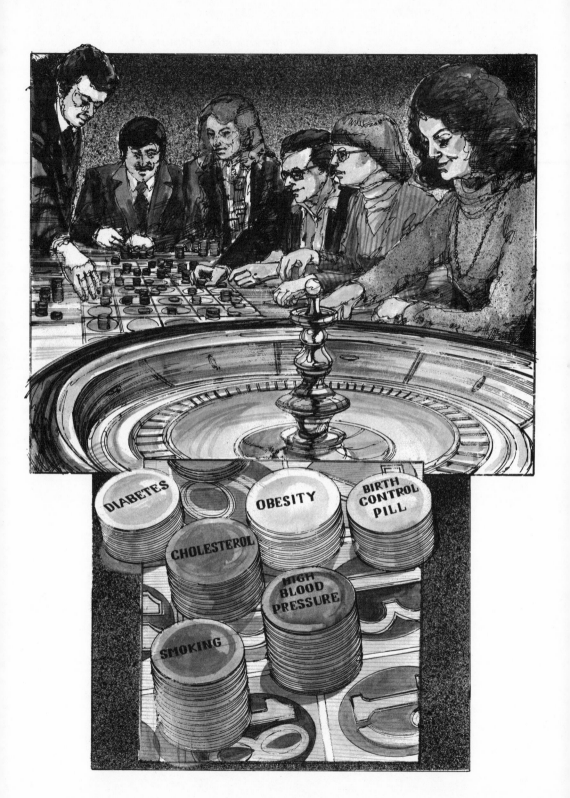

12

Taking Risks:
Your Habits Matter

HEART DISEASE is as American as apple pie. Or maybe we should say as American as bacon and eggs.

We have one of the highest rates of heart disease in the world (Finland is higher), and this is not without reason. To a large degree it is because of the way we live. While we often act as though our habits don't matter, it is clear that they do. And some of these habits drastically increase the risk of heart disease. To paraphrase one book title that says it all, THE AMERICAN WAY OF LIFE MAY BE HAZARDOUS TO YOUR HEALTH.

Risk factors are conditions that contribute to the development of cardiovascular disease. There are two kinds of risks—controllable and noncontrollable.

Noncontrollable Risks

Among the risks you can't control are your age, your sex, and your heredity. Coronary disease becomes more common as people grow older, it is more common among men than women—at least until women reach the menopause—and it is more common among people whose close relatives have

67

had cardiovascular disease, especially so, if they had it at a young age. O.K., you can't do anything about that. What can you control?

Controllable Risks

Among the risk factors that *you* can do something about are: high blood pressure, cigarette smoking, cholesterol intake, excess weight, inactivity, diabetes, and a few other things we'll go over.

By far and away, the most important risk factors, according to a major study in Framingham, Massachusetts, are:

- Cigarette smoking

- High blood pressure

- High cholesterol.

These are such powerful risks they are often termed the "Big Three." And all of these risks can add up. Leaving more than one risk factor uncontrolled is a considerably bigger gamble than leaving just a single one.

Note from the chart on the next page that if you have high cholesterol *and* high blood pressure *and* smoke cigarettes, you're really taking a chance. The risk of heart attack for someone who has all these characteristics as opposed to someone who has none of them is *five times* higher.

And if you have a family history of cardiovascular disease, this may be because you or your relatives tend to have high cholesterol or high blood pressure, so that a so-called non-controllable risk, heredity, may in fact be within your control.

Some people think that coffee is a risk, but several studies have failed to show convincingly that coffee drinking has harmful effects on the cardiovascular system.

DIABETES: ANOTHER RISK   Are you possibly a diabetic? If you have been hospitalized with a heart condition, your doctor has probably determined whether you are or aren't. If you don't know, try the questionnaire on page 70.

The Risk of Having a Heart Attack If You Have High Blood Pressure, Smoke Cigarettes, and Have a High Cholesterol Level—The "Big Three" Risk Factors

Risk

5 times

3 times

1½ times

No high blood pressure, high cholesterol, or cigarettes

Cigarettes

High cholesterol and cigarettes

High blood pressure, high cholesterol, and cigarettes

Source: Extrapolated from American Heart Association data, based on the Framingham, Mass. Heart Study.

Diabetes is a remarkably silent disease, and this is important: *One of two people with diabetes doesn't even realize he or she has it.*

Thus, maybe you're a diabetic and don't know it. Check with your physician to be sure.

Are You a Possible Diabetic?

Take 30 seconds to answer the questions on this check-list:

	YES	NO
1. Any diabetics in your family?	☐	☐
2. Are you over 40?	☐	☐
3. Are you overweight?	☐	☐
4. Any sudden weight loss?	☐	☐
5. Are you constantly thirsty?	☐	☐
6. Do you overeat?	☐	☐
7. Do you urinate too frequently?	☐	☐
8. Do you tire easily?	☐	☐
9. Do your wounds heal slowly?	☐	☐
10. Any tingling, numbness, or pains in your fingers or toes?	☐	☐
11. Any changes in vision?	☐	☐
12. Does your skin itch frequently?	☐	☐
13. Women: have you had a baby weighing over nine pounds at birth?	☐	☐

Interpretation: Every "yes" answer to the above quiz raises the possibility of your being a diabetic.

What is diabetes? It's a disorder in which the body does not make proper use of sugar, so that there is too much sugar in the bloodstream and the body therefore runs less efficiently.

People who have diabetes have a much greater chance of developing coronary disease—and of developing it when they are young—as well as having stroke, blindness, kidney disorders, and vessel diseases in the legs.

If you think diabetes is uncommon, that's not true. It strikes 5 percent of the population—6 million Americans a year. It most often develops in persons over 40; however, since it runs in families, even youngsters can get it.

Diabetes can be checked with proper exercise, by eating the right amounts of foods at the right time, and, if necessary, with insulin administration, although most adults with diabetes don't need insulin.

THE PILL   Another risk factor that you can control is birth-control pills, which have been linked to the early development of heart attack, stroke, and high blood pressure. In addition, these pills may cause inflammation of the veins of the legs, a disease called *thrombophlebitis.* This condition in turn can be the cause of another disease called *pulmonary embolism,* which may result when a blood clot formed in a vein breaks off and travels in the bloodstream to a lung, where it blocks an artery.

Women on birth-control pills have a severalfold greater likelihood of having heart attacks than do women not on the pill. Furthermore, oral contraceptives may *add* to the risk produced by other factors such as cigarette smoking, high blood pressure, or high cholesterol levels. Thus, if one or more of these is present in your life and you take birth-control pills besides, your chances of suffering a coronary or stroke go up even higher.

So what do we recommend about birth-control pills? First of all, no one, not even a healthy person, should take them without checking with her doctor. While it's probably O.K. for young women to take them for awhile, if you are over 35 or 40 or have some of the other risk factors in your life or, of course, if you have already suffered a heart attack or stroke, oral contraceptives are best avoided.

But remember, you must weigh all these facts against the risk of pregnancy itself.

Evaluating Your Chances

The table on the following page is not magical, is not a scientifically proven means of accurately estimating one's chances for developing cardiovascular disease. However, at least it gives you some ball-park idea of where you stand. We urge you to grab a pencil and take a moment to determine what

Cardiovascular Disease (CD) Risk Calculator

NONCONTROLLABLE RISK FACTORS

Heredity	No family history	1–2 close relatives (parent or sibling develop CD over age 60)	1–2 close relatives (parent or sibling develop CD under age 60)
Sex	Female (premenopausal)	—	Male or postmenopausal female
Age	10–20	21–40	41–50

CONTROLLABLE RISK FACTORS

Controllable with physician's help

Blood pressure (systolic)	Under 120	120–139	140–159
Diabetes	No	—	—

Controllable with self-help

Cigarettes	No	Inhaled pipe or cigars	Under ½ pack per day
Blood cholesterol	Under 170	170–199	200–219
Body weight	Under standard	Standard	5–15 lb. over
Exercise	Vigorous (job or recreational)	Active (job or recreation)	—
SCORE	0	1	2

3	4	5	6
Several relatives (including aunts or uncles; some develop CD under age 55)	—	—	—
—	—	—	—
Over 50	—	—	—
160–179	180–199	200–229	Over 230
Yes	—	—	—
½–1 pack per day	—	1–2 packs per day	Over 2 packs per day
220–239	240–269	270–299	Over 300
16–25 lb. over	26–50 lb. over	More than 50 lb. over	—
Sedentary	—	—	—
3	4	5	6

YOUR SCORE	YOUR RISK PROFILE
Under 10	Very low
10–14	Low
15–20	Moderately increased
21–24	High
Over 25	Very high

your risk profile is. For each risk factor, select the statement that most closely fits you, and then add the score located at the bottom of each column. Your total score then provides an estimate of your risk of developing cardiovascular problems.

After you've completed your profile, read those of Chapters 13 through 19 that seem to apply to you, to see how you can manage these risk factors.

13

Stress

THERE IS AN INTERESTING phenomenon as regards this "risk factor." Public-opinion surveys show that Americans believe *stress* is the most important cause of coronary heart disease—more important, in fact, than high blood pressure, smoking, or diet. The popularity of this idea is no doubt one of the reasons why so many people don't pay attention to these other risk factors. (They also get little in the way of good advice from the advertising by the tobacco, dairy, and egg industries.)

But does stress really contribute to heart disease? A few physicians assert that the trials and tribulations of modern life—job pressures, family squabbles, money problems, illness of a relative, for example—add up to a big risk factor. Others say the problem is internal; it is how strongly you personally react to outside annoyances and pressures that determines your liability.

Type A Behavior?

Indeed, some investigators have gone so far as to classify two types of behavior, Type A and Type B. Type A personalities

75

are competitive, hard-driving individuals, both at work and at play. They are constantly concerned about time and are easily irritated, so that when they are caught behind a slow driver or made to wait in a restaurant, for example, they begin to boil inside. The Type B person, by contrast, is calmer and more relaxed, able to take life as it comes. Of course, the latter type, it is thought by these investigators, is less apt to get a heart attack.

What do we think of all this? We are skeptical. The reports linking stress or behavior type to risk are too scanty. They have not been sufficiently corroborated by other independent investigators working in the same field. One problem, for example, has been the difficulty in accurately measuring each person's "stress score." And certainly classifying people as being either Type A or Type B seems to be an oversimplification: everybody has traits on both sides of the fence. We are not Type A *or* Type B; we are a little of each.

Moreover, studies of life-styles in various cultures do not confirm the stress hypothesis. Some peoples live and work amongst crowded, competitive, time-urgent conditions, yet their rate of coronary disease is extremely low. By contrast, some of the highest rates in the world have been found among Finnish loggers and farmers, who lead quiet outdoor lives. Finally, a great amount of atherosclerotic disease was found among a group of American railroad workers who had apparently adapted well to a paternalistic, friendly employer and were not living in a state of struggle and time urgency. In short, there is going to have to be more research on the subject of stress before we can conclude that it is a true coronary risk.

Cues

A number of cues suggest you're having difficulty handling stress. See if any of these fit:

• Constant agitation

• Failing to finish what you've started

- Inability to concentrate. Does your mind wander aimlessly?

- Muscular tensions, tying you in knots

- Feelings of uncertainty or vulnerability

- Nervous gestures such as grinding your teeth or nail biting

- Sleeplessness

- Feeling low

Détente

Stress is universal. Nothing is going to make it disappear entirely. So why not face it squarely. Why not accept life for what it is and learn to coexist with its inevitable pressures. It's much as if you were going to walk out into a snowstorm: you know very well you can't change the weather, so you simply prepare for it and carry on. Here are a few tips that may help you deal with stress:

- Know what makes you tick, those habitual ways you react to life's tribulations.

- Be aware of your needs—of what really counts.

- Stay with the here and now, rather than worrying about the future or lamenting the past; take one thing at a time.

- Avoid, or at least minimize, unnecessary competitive, or aggressive interactions.

- Set aside quiet time for yourself once or twice daily—an opportunity to still your body and your mind.

- Learn some relaxation exercises. There are many books, tapes, and classes that address these.

- Use visualization. Create healthy and peaceful pictures in your mind to replace those noxious, negative thoughts.

- Get out of situations that are clearly untenable.

- Lighten up and savor life.

In making your comeback, you know that some things will probably have to change as far as diet, exercise, and the like. While you are revising your behavior in those areas, it makes sense to revise it in the area of stress, too. Stress, after all, is what makes a lot of people smoke too much, drink too much, and eat too much—and *those* factors may very well contribute to coronary problems. There will always be problems and pressures, of course, but at least you can begin to make a pact with yourself that you won't get lost in overreacting next time you get behind a slow truck on a mountain road or can't catch your waiter's eye. Life is better when it is calmer.

Your Stress Profile

To get an idea how much external stress you have in your life, try taking the following quiz. *But let's be honest, the real stress comes from inside—from your response to all these external adversities that life throws at you.*

Testing Your Life Stresses

Which of the following have you had within the last two years? Circle the number on the right.

LIFE EVENT	MEAN VALUE
1. Death of spouse	100
2. Divorce	73
3. Marital separation from mate	65
4. Detention in jail or other institution	63
5. Death of a close family member	63
6. Major personal injury or illness	53
7. Marriage	50
8. Being fired at work	47
9. Marital reconciliation with mate	45
10. Retirement from work	45
11. Major change in the health or behavior of a family member	44
12. Pregnancy	40
13. Sexual difficulties	39
14. Gaining a new family member (e.g., through birth, adoption, oldster moving in, etc.)	39
15. Major business readjustment (e.g., merger, reorganization, bankruptcy, etc.)	39
16. Major change in financial state (e.g., a lot worse off or a lot better off than usual)	38
17. Death of a close friend	37
18. Changing to a different line of work	36
19. Major change in the number of arguments with spouse (e.g., either a lot more or a lot less than usual regarding child-rearing, personal habits, etc.)	35
20. Taking on a mortgage greater than $10,000 (e.g., purchasing a home, business, etc.)	31
21. Foreclosure on a mortgage or loan	30
22. Major changes in responsibilities at work (e.g., promotion, demotion, lateral transfer)	29
23. Son or daughter leaving home (e.g., marriage, attending college, etc.)	29
24. In-law troubles	29

25. Outstanding personal achievement | 28
26. Wife beginning or ceasing work outside the home | 26
27. Beginning or ceasing formal schooling | 26
28. Major change in living conditions (e.g., building a new home, remodeling, deterioration of home or neighborhood) | 25
29. Revision of personal habits (dress, manners, associations, etc.) | 24
30. Troubles with the boss | 23
31. Major change in working hours or conditions | 20
32. Change in residence | 20
33. Changing to a new school | 20
34. Major change in usual type and/or amount of recreation | 19
35. Major change in church activities (e.g., a lot more or a lot less than usual) | 19
36. Major change in social activities (e.g., clubs, dancing, movies, visiting, etc.) | 18
37. Taking on a mortgage or loan less than $10,000 (e.g., purchasing a car, TV, freezer, etc.) | 17
38. Major change in sleeping habits (a lot more or a lot less sleep, or change in part of day when asleep) | 16
39. Major change in number of family get-togethers (e.g., a lot more or a lot less than usual) | 15
40. Major change in eating habits (a lot more or a lot less food intake, or very different meal hours or surroundings) | 15
41. Vacation | 13
42. Christmas | 12
43. Minor violations of the law (e.g., traffic tickets, jaywalking, disturbing the peace, etc.) | 11

Total score: _____

Interpretation:

0–149	Low stress
150–199	Mild stress
200–299	Moderate stress
300 or more	Major stress

Source: T. H. Holmes and R. H. Rahe, "The Social Readjustment Rating Scale," *Journal of Psychosomatic Research* II (1967): 213–18.

14

High Blood Pressure

MANY PEOPLE THINK they can tell high blood pressure is present by headaches or other symptoms, but the only way to know if you've got it is to have it measured—with a pressure cuff attached to a measuring device called a sphygmomanometer (*sfig-mo-mah-NOM-e-ter*), which describes the blood pressure in terms of two numbers: *systolic* and *diastolic*.

Systolic pressure (the first number) is a measure of the tension on the artery walls caused by the beating heart pumping blood into the arteries.

Diastolic pressure is a measure of the tension remaining between heartbeats.

The average blood pressure reading for adults is about 120 systolic and 80 diastolic. This is called "120 over 80" and is generally written "120/80." Blood pressure varies somewhat, depending on activity. Usually, it is lower when you're at rest and higher when you're active, excited, or under stress. Normal blood pressure under relaxed conditions should be below 140/90, but 160/95 is probably acceptable in people in their 70s and over.

However, when blood pressure goes up and *stays there,* the condition is called *hypertension* or "high blood pressure."

Hypertension should not be confused with "nervousness," a hyperactive personality, or with a blushing complexion. It simply means high pressure within the artery.

High blood pressure is extraordinarily common, affecting 55 million adults in the United States—that's 1 in 5. And it usually appears without producing *any* symptoms. Where do you stand? The chart below shows the chances of having a heart attack depending on one's *systolic* blood pressure.

In most cases, the cause of hypertension is unknown, though occasionally abnormalities of the kidneys, the blood vessels feeding them, or certain substances in the bloodstream may be at fault. High blood pressure also runs in families, so if one of your parents had it, there is a chance you can develop it, too.

High blood pressure occurs when the walls of the small arteries clamp down excessively on the blood that flows by, thereby raising the pressure. The danger of this is that, over

The Risk of Having a Heart Attack If You Have High Blood Pressure

A person whose blood pressure at systole (when the heart contracts) is over 150 has more than two times the risk of heart attack of a person with systolic blood pressure under 120.

Source: Extrapolated from American Heart Association data, based on the Framingham, Mass., Heart Study.

the years, this excessive pressure can wear out the arteries and overwork the heart and, if not treated, can lead to atherosclerosis, strokes, coronary artery disease, congestive heart failure, visual difficulties, and diseases of the kidneys. It can also aggravate angina pectoris by increasing the severity and frequency of the pain. Hypertension seldom disappears entirely.

The good news is that hypertension is dangerous only when it is ignored or inadequately treated, and in most cases it can be well controlled.

Treatment

It takes two to tackle high blood pressure—you and your doctor. *Dieting* to take off that excess weight, often with the aid of an *exercise program,* represents one means of correcting hypertension. *Medication* and *restriction of salt intake* are the two other principal approaches. You can often get by without medication if your blood pressure is only slightly high. And since risks add up, why not control cholesterol and smoking too?

It may be possible for the physician to lower your blood pressure by prescribing only a single medication (usually in pill form), but on occasion the dose of that pill has to be raised to two or more tablets daily, and combinations of two, three, or even four different drugs are sometimes needed to bring the pressure down. A number of medications, called *antihypertensives,* lower the blood pressure; these are often given with *diuretics,* medicines that rid the body of excessive fluid and salt and drop the pressure. The medications used to treat hypertension are described in detail in Appendix A.

The medications that are given to help bring the blood pressure down *must be taken regularly,* as frequently as prescribed by your physician, since failure to do so generally results in the blood pressure returning to its previously high levels. This is very important. The biggest difficulty with treating high blood pressure is that patients don't take their medications, don't understand them, miss doses, or get sick of (or from) them and then discontinue them. Not following the prescription *exactly* remains the major problem in the treatment of high blood pressure.

Another problem is that many of the drugs used to treat high blood pressure have *side effects,* which vary greatly in their severity and frequency from one person to another. What will happen is that your doctor will start you on a medication and, if it produces bothersome symptoms, will switch you to another drug. Thus, treatment of high blood pressure involves some trial and error.

A Salty Thought

You can also do a great deal for yourself in the treatment of hypertension, and that is to cut down on the amount of salt (sodium) you eat. Although salt is frequently mentioned in diets prepared for heart patients, it is *not* a particularly important factor in the control of coronary disease, and too many people get put on a low-salt diet who don't need it. However, high blood pressure and congestive heart failure are the two conditions where it is desirable, often mandatory, to restrict the use of salt in the diet. The reason is that salt holds onto water, overfilling the arteries and veins with water, and thus further raising the blood pressure. It can also produce swelling of the ankles or abdomen and congestion within the lungs in patients with congestive heart failure.

Although we said some people get put on low-salt diets who shouldn't be, the fact remains that Americans eat an incredible amount of salt, far more than is good for them. *We should all cut back to some degree on our salt consumption.* Foods particularly high in salt are:

- *Meats*—certain meats such as ham, bacon, sausage, lunch meats, hot dogs, corned beef, anchovies, smoked fish.

- *Cured vegetables*—certain vegetables such as french fries, potato chips, salted nuts, popcorn, pickles, relishes, olives, sauerkraut.

- *Soups*—bouillon and canned soups.

- *Condiments*—mustard, catsup, relishes, Worcestershire sauce, horseradish.

- *Other*—commercial salad dressings, party spreads and dips, pretzels, crackers, baking powder, certain cheeses, monosodium glutamate—even softened water.

Certain drugs also contain sodium, such as the alkalizers you take for stomach upset (bicarbonate of soda and Alka-Seltzer).

And if you chew tobacco, you should know it is high in sodium.

The best approach to limiting your salt is:

- Don't automatically salt your food at the table.

- When cooking, flavor with spices other than salt.

- Minimize those foods highest in salt content, especially processed and fast foods. If you can see it (the salt, that is), don't eat it.

- If your physician O.K.'s it, you may use a salt substitute.

Use your common sense here, even though, we're told, it's the least common of all the senses.

15

Smoking: Playing with Fire

LET'S SAY YOU'RE a young or middle-aged woman and healthy, with no blood-pressure problems or other disorders. Your main vice is that you smoke—say, about two packs of cigarettes a day. If so, you are *two to three times* more apt to have a heart attack than a nonsmoker, and there's a fifty-fifty chance it could be fatal.

And, of course, we haven't even mentioned lung, throat, or tongue cancer; bronchitis; emphysema; stroke; and other disorders caused by cigarettes. The fact is, if you smoke two or more packs a day, you are essentially trading a minute of life for a minute of smoking. Life insurance companies know this, or they wouldn't offer reductions in premiums for nonsmokers. The U.S. Secretary of Health and Human Services has called smoking "slow-motion suicide." And as the surgeon general has put it, "Cigarette smoking should be considered the most important of the known modifiable risk factors" (see the chart on the next page).

Let's face a few more sobering facts:

- If you smoke, your risk of a heart attack triples.

The Risk of Having a Heart Attack
If You Smoke Cigarettes

A person who smokes more than a pack of cigarettes a day has nearly twice the risk of heart attack of a nonsmoker.

Source: Extrapolated from American Heart Association data, based on the Framingham, Mass., Heart Study.

- If you've already had a myocardial infarction, and keep smoking, your chance of surviving another one is less.

- Smoking contributes to 350,000 fatalities in the U.S. annually, at an estimated cost to the nation of $37 billion.

- Cigarette smoke is the single most toxic substance people put into their bodies, and it so pollutes the atmosphere as to affect innocent bystanders as well.

- Thirty to 40 percent of the fatalities from coronary disease are attributable to cigarettes.

The way cigarettes bring on heart damage is still something of a mystery, but three possible explanations are:

- The nicotine repeatedly overstimulates the heart and makes it more irritable.

- The carbon monoxide absorbed into your blood takes the place of oxygen and hampers nourishment of the heart muscle and other tissues. People with angina pectoris develop the chest pain quicker if they smoke. Even being in the same room with people who are smoking may aggravate these chest pains.

- The smoke damages the lining of the coronary arteries, allowing artery-clogging cholesterol and other debris to build up and narrow the passageways.

Jekyll and Hyde

The good news, however, is the phenomenally rapid benefit that results from stopping smoking: the risk of coronary attacks drops by half in the first year. And 5 to 10 years after you quit smoking you are statistically no more at risk than someone like you with a similar problem but who has never smoked.

Our intent is not to lecture you but to help you quit. There is no doubt that it can be difficult, though some people seem to be able to quit "cold turkey" and just suddenly give up smoking for good. The first thing that is required is *motivation.* You've got to want to do it. And the motivation must be *positive:* think how good you're going to feel, how nice the air will smell, how far and fast you will be able to run or swim. Accentuate the positive.

If you are motivated, then you have to make the decision to quit. You have to *choose* —and if you continue smoking, you should realize you are in effect choosing that smoking is more worthwhile than quitting. Have a Dr. Jekyll/Mr. Hyde debate with yourself, stating all the reasons for quitting versus not quitting.

Quitting Tips

If you have decided to quit, here are some hints; be a quitter for once.

- Set a date to stop and do it, completely!
- Be aware you will be uncomfortable for a week. However,

it's O.K. to be uncomfortable. You won't suffer unbearable pain, you're not going to die from it, and the discomfort won't last. The physiological addiction, the nicotine in the body, probably lasts only 72 hours or so. Thereafter, you'll have a psychological desire to smoke; that is, a desire stemming from memories of pleasure in enjoying the cigarettes. And this desire may last, who knows how long.

- As you quit smoking, your "nervous appetite" may increase, but remember this is really your desire for cigarettes in disguise. Face up to the fact. In all likelihood, if you're able to stop smoking, you're able to watch your diet, too.

- Understand that stopping smoking is a *learned skill,* just as is learning to play the violin, tennis, and so on. Thus, you can *learn* to live without cigarettes and *learn* not to crave them.

- For a few days keep a diary so you can become *aware* of when and where you smoke, and for what reasons. You will probably find there are patterns in your smoking, so you can start to do something about modifying them. If you are aware that what you really want is a cigarette, you won't necessarily end up eating that extra piece of pie (thinking erroneously it was the dessert you wanted).

- Get *moral support* by making an agreement with a friend to quit at the same time. (But, beware: if your friend goes back to smoking, this could be used as an excuse by you to do the same.)

- Don't set yourself up for failure. People ask themselves, "What will happen if I become too nervous?" "What if the family gets mad at me if I fail?" "What if I start eating too much?" Many people are afraid they won't be able to work or get through the day or that they will want a cigarette so badly they will be unable to resist. Anticipating these fears makes it easier to deal with them. And don't be discouraged if you have tried but failed in stopping smoking in the past. Everyone learns something from their past attempts that gives them ammunition the next time.

Groups to Help You Quit

Many people can stop smoking on willpower alone, but if you have trouble, don't fight it. Various stop-smoking clinics and other organizations are listed under "Smokers Information and Treatment Centers" in the Yellow Pages of the phone book. Or you may want to contact your local heart association or lung society for recommendations. To an extent, each method or clinic has been successful in getting some people to quit, but none has been demonstrated to work for all smokers. One of the great values of these groups is they provide reinforcement and support in the months and years to come if the old urge to smoke hangs on.

Among the more prominent methods are the following:

- *Some clinics stress a commonsense, positive approach*—in which the importance of motivation and the good that will come out of quitting is emphasized, and in which you are shown how life can go on as before—but without cigarettes.

- *Behavior modification*—in which another, more desirable activity (chewing gum, drawing, or whatever) is *substituted* for the smoking. This method teaches you to avoid situations where you know you will want to smoke (for example, with coffee or while driving or sitting at the table after dinner) and to avoid carrying cigarettes or to carry them in an inconvenient place.

- *Hypnosis*—can be a valuable adjunct to quitting, although it can't make you quit. It can strengthen your determination, and it may make you more comfortable during the immediate withdrawal period. It is seldom effective alone, but is most helpful when combined with a planned smoking cessation program.

- *Aversion therapy*—in which an undesirable stimulus such as rapidly puffing on cigarettes is used to discourage you from smoking. A variation is to have you smoke in a small, poorly ventilated space to the point where it becomes unpleasant.

- *Scare or fear therapy* —in which the risks are vividly demonstrated with pictures or real-life examples of patients with serious diseases that result from long-term smoking. This approach is seldom valuable when used alone, although certainly everyone should be well informed as to the potential hazards of smoking cigarettes.

- *Nicotine containing gum* —helps some people get through those first few weeks, but it, too, can be habit forming.

Still, we understand that quitting cigarettes is not easy, and you should feel free to explore any method that seems workable to you.

One last point: There is no such thing as a safe cigarette. Though some people switch to low tar and nicotine cigarettes, they end up smoking twice as many as before. And neither these nor the special filter cigarettes cut down your risk.

Remember that *you* hold the key to success. Either alone or with professional assistance, you must begin to deal with the stresses in your life without smoking—by understanding yourself and by believing that you truly can pull it off. Success won't last unless you keep working at it and want it to last.

16

Fat City: Cholesterol, Saturated Fats, Triglycerides

AMERICANS EAT more meat per capita than people do in any European country, and only in countries with vast grazing lands such as New Zealand and Argentina is the consumption greater.

Now, although this habit might seem to date back to the American legend of cowboys and cattle drives, it is an interesting fact that up until 10 or so years ago meat consumption was up *40 percent* over what it had been in the early 1900s—when the Wild West began to disappear. During that time there had also been a dramatic rise in the amount of fat consumed—up to 25 percent. But in the last 10 to 20 years, folks have become more sensible about their diets and we've begun to see a fall off in this trend.

By "fat" we do not mean that stuff that, unfortunately, seems to accumulate around the waist and hips of so many of us. Here we mean *blood fats*.

There are two kinds of blood fats that are associated with cardiovascular disease and heart attack: *cholesterol* (the one that's grabbed all the headlines) and *triglycerides*. Cholesterol in particular, according to the preponderance of present

medical opinion, is thought to contribute to the development of atherosclerosis, so we'll describe it first.

Cholesterol

Cholesterol is a fatlike substance found in the blood and tissues and is essential to the body function. A certain amount of it is necessary to maintain the body in proper working order, but in excess it deposits in artery linings and narrows the vessels.

How do you know if you have an excessive amount of cholesterol in your blood? A simple blood test is the only way to tell. Then compare your cholesterol level with the chart below to ascertain your risk.

Throughout the world, those peoples that consume foods containing large amounts of cholesterol and saturated fats tend on average to run higher levels of blood cholesterol and therefore, to develop cardiovascular problems more commonly. And populations from countries that eat foods low in these substances have lower blood cholesterol and are relatively free of coronary disease.

It is becoming clear from a number of national studies that by decreasing your blood cholesterol you lower the risk of developing, or dying from, coronary disease. And, equally exciting, people who already have coronary disease and successfully lower their cholesterol are considerably less likely to have further narrowing of their coronary vessels.

The American Heart Association recommends a daily cholesterol intake of no more than 250 milligrams, and only 30 percent of the calories we eat should contain fat—10 percent of this being saturated fat and 10 percent polyunsaturated.

The Light and Dark Sides of Cholesterol

Because oil and water don't mix, cholesterol is carried through the blood by a special transport system called *lipoproteins* (LDL, low-density lipoprotein, and HDL, high-density lipoprotein). When cholesterol is carried along by LDL, it may be deposited

The Risk of Having a Heart Attack If You Have a High Cholesterol Level

A person with a blood cholesterol measurement of 250 or above has about two and a half times the risk of heart attack as one with cholesterol below 194. The higher the blood cholesterol, the greater the risk of heart attack and cardiovascular disease.

Source: Extrapolated from American Heart Association data, based on the Framingham, Mass. Heart Study.

into the walls of the artery and produce coronary narrowing. Thus, a high LDL-cholesterol increases a person's risk of coronary disease. Diets rich in cholesterol raise the LDL-cholesterol, and a high LDL also runs in some families.

In contrast, another transporter, HDL, may actually remove cholesterol from artery walls, and a high amount of HDL-cholesterol in the blood protects against heart attack. HDL-cholesterol levels may be raised—to your benefit—by stopping smoking, losing weight, exercising, and by moderate consumption of alcohol—at most one or two drinks a day (beer, highballs, or wine).

How can you reduce your cholesterol level? By avoiding, as we shall show, two kinds of foods: (1) foods high in *cholesterol*, and (2) foods high in *saturated fats*, because the body manufactures cholesterol from these fats.

When we say "avoid" these foods, by the way, we don't mean you must never again have a steak or an ice cream cone. As we said back in the chapter on doctor's orders versus doctor's recommendations, our dietary advice need not be followed rigidly. Any food may be eaten on occasion without harm—it's O.K. to have a thick steak when you're dining out on your anniversary, say. But we do recommend that you try and avoid *repeatedly* eating foods high in cholesterol and saturated fats, and learn which foods are best to substitute for those fatty ones.

Foods High in Cholesterol and Saturated Fats

In decreasing order (highest first), these foods are high in cholesterol and saturated fats.

- Egg yolk
- Organ meat
- Dairy products—cheese, whole milk, cream, cream cheese, ice cream, and butter
- Hydrogenated fats and oils—including animal fats (beef, pork, and chicken fats), lard or shortening
- Some red meats—such as pork, beef, and processed meats
- Duck and goose
- Other red meats—such as lamb and veal
- Shrimp and prawns

Let's look at each of these groups.

EGGS.   Egg yolks are the single greatest source of cholesterol in the American diet. By and large, avoid them, including dishes containing eggs and foods such as egg noodles and egg breads.

Suggestion: Eat all the egg whites you wish (they contain no cholesterol). When cooking, substitute two egg whites where one egg yolk is called for. Egg substitutes are also available. Try the different brands until you find one you like.

ORGAN MEAT.   All meats (including poultry and fish) contain some cholesterol, but organ meats such as liver, kidney, tongue, heart, brain, and sweetbreads contain huge amounts. Have them on special occasions but otherwise avoid.

CHEESE.   Since most cheeses are made from whole milk, they are high in saturated fat. Avoid Brie, Camembert, cheddar, Monterey, Muenster, Roquefort, and Swiss. Especially avoid eating large quantities of cheese.
Suggestion: Serve cheeses made from nonfat or partially skimmed milk: bakers' cheese, cottage cheese, farmer's cheese, Mozzarella, sapsago, and low-fat parmesan.

WHOLE MILK.   Whole milk is high in saturated fats. Low-fat milk contains about half the amount of fat. Nonfat has very little such fat.
Suggestion: Drink nonfat milk (and occasionally low-fat milk) instead of whole milk. Buttermilk is also acceptable.

DAIRY CREAMS.   Since these are high in saturated fats, avoid all, including whipping cream, dessert cream, and half-and-half.
Suggestion: Substitute nondairy creamers (but not those made from coconut oil). For recipes requiring cream or sour cream, you may substitute a nonfat yogurt, low-fat milk, or buttermilk.

ICE CREAM.   Save for special occasions.
Suggestion: Serve ice milk or, preferably, sherbert, sorbet, or Weight Watchers Frozen Desserts.

BUTTER.   Avoid.
Suggestion: Substitute polyunsaturated margarines (in either small tubs or cubes) made from safflower, corn, soybean, or cottonseed oil. Check the labels, and use only those margarines in which the first ingredient listed shows a *liquid* oil. Avoid those that show "hydrogenated" or "partially hydrogenated" oils among the first listed ingredients, since they contain more saturated fats than the polyunsaturated margarines do. The next section explains this point.

COOKING FATS AND OILS. Certain vegetable oils such as palm and coconut oil are also high in saturated fats, as is chocolate.

A special word about *polyunsaturated fats*, which are found in vegetable oils: These do not convert into cholesterol. Indeed, they actually *lower* the amount of cholesterol in your bloodstream. The polyunsaturated fats best for you, in order of preference, are: safflower, sunflower, corn, soybean, and cottonseed.

Polyunsaturated fats are usually liquid at room temperature. But in manufacturing they may undergo "hardening" or "hydrogenation," which makes them more solid and therefore higher in saturated fat. Thus, avoid oils described on labels as "saturated," "hardened," "hydrogenated," or "partially hydrogenated." You will find these in certain peanut butters, shortening, whipped toppings, salad dressings, hydrogenated margarines, and processed bakery products.

Suggestions: When cooking:

• Substitute polyunsaturated oils for saturated cooking and salad oils.

• Deep-fry foods only in polyunsaturated oils, and don't reuse the oils or they will become saturated.

• Instead of using chocolate (which is high in saturated fat) in recipes, use cocoa powder mixed with nonfat milk.

CONVENIENCE FOODS. Potato chips (except the polyunsaturated ones) and other fried foods, meats, and TV dinners; many cake mixes, cookies, donuts, sweetrolls, butter rolls, and muffins; and similar types of commercially available processed foods are high in saturated fat. Nuts, however, are O.K., except for cashews and macadamia nuts (which are high in saturated fats), but regardless of the type of fats nuts contain, they are high in calories.

RED MEAT. All of the red meats—beef, pork, lamb, and veal—contain saturated fat, which can be seen along the edges of the meat and as part of the marbling within the center. The saturated fats are greater in "prime" cuts than "choice," and least in "good" qualities. In general, pork (especially bacon and spareribs) contains more saturated fats and veal less, compared to the other red meats. Cholesterol is found not just in the fatty portion of the meat but also lies invisible in the lean muscles; so the more meat you eat, the more cholesterol.

Other meats high in saturated fats are hamburger (ground round having the least—have your butcher trim and grind to order), smoked meats, and mutton.

Suggestion: Serve red meats only 1 or 2 times a week, using modest portions (approximately 1/3 pound or 5 1/2 oz. for active working men, 1/4 pound or 4 oz. for smaller and less active people). Serving up the meat on smaller plates is often helpful from a psychological standpoint. Select only the lean cuts, trim off as much fat as possible, and cook by broiling, barbecuing, roasting, or pan frying, so that the fat is allowed to run off.

PREPARED MEATS. Almost all processed meats—hot dogs, salami, liverwurst, bologna, sausage—contain not only large amounts of saturated fat but also a lot of salt. Serve as infrequently as possible.

STEWS, SOUP, AND CHILI. Avoid eating any broth or stock that has just been prepared from animal meat. Refrigerate overnight and then skim off the fat that has moved to the top.

SHRIMP. It's O.K. to eat shrimp or prawns, but sparingly. Be aware that it is the shellfish that contains the highest amount of cholesterol.

Triglycerides

We've talked about Cholesterol and its sidekick, Saturated Fats. Now let's talk about that other blood fat, triglycerides.

These are substances that may be associated with cardiovascular disease, although the evidence is not as clear on this point as it is on cholesterol.

Excess triglycerides may appear in four situations: inheritance of the trait (though triglycerides often don't become a problem unless one is overweight also), obesity (from consuming too many calories), excess alcohol consumption, and diabetes.

How do you know if you have too many triglycerides in your blood? As with cholesterol, a simple blood test will give your physician the information. If he or she finds your triglyceride level too high, you will probably be asked to: lose weight, start an exercise program, reduce your sugar intake, and cut down on the wine and spirits. In subsequent chapters we'll tell you how to handle those suggestions.

Delectable and Nourishing Meals

Even if you have high cholesterol levels, note that we aren't asking you to live on rye bread and grapefruit alone. And note also that you can eat *any* food occasionally. Most of your meals, however, can easily be made delicious and kept healthy with a number of "natural, unprocessed" foods. Some ideas:

- *Fish:* This has virtually no saturated fat. Eat it as often as you like. Shellfish (except for shrimp) is also good, and can be eaten at least 2 or 3 times a week.

  Fish and shellfish contain a type of fat called *Omega,* which tends to protect against heart attack; the fatter the fish the more the Omega. But don't take fish oil capsules unless your doctor recommends them.

- *Poultry:* Eat chicken and turkey, being sure to trim the skin and its fatty underlayer before cooking. However, avoid duck and goose, and the chicken's giblets, liver, and gizzard, since they're high in saturated fat.

- *Whole grain breads, cereals, grains*

- *Pasta and rice*

- *All the fresh fruits and vegetables you want*

- *Beans, lentils, legumes*

And if you're worried about not getting enough protein, because of having to cut down on meat and milk, you might try even more whole grains, legumes, beans, and soybean products such as tofu.

Expanding Your Culinary Horizons

If you're locked into the typical American meat-and-potatoes regimen, now's your chance to find out what the rest of the world offers. Here are some places to look for foods low in cholesterol and saturated fats: different spices, herbs, vinegars, flavorings that don't add cholesterol; Chinese or Japanese cooking; Central American and Latin American food; Middle Eastern cuisine; North African cuisine. However, be careful of the type and amount of fat the recipe calls for. Both olive and peanut oil are used in many cultures and these contain a type of fat we haven't mentioned—monounsaturated fat—this one, also, is relatively safe.

In exploring such areas, you'll be doing your family a favor, too. After all, our eating patterns are usually established when we are young. If you would like your children to avoid some of the things you've been through, perhaps you can start them down a different culinary path through your example. And, of course, the modifications in your diet become easier for you if everyone in the family is sharing them with you.

Check the appendixes at the end of the book. They offer valuable information to help you with your shopping and other food-related matters.

The Future

Will all this changing of diet prevent coronary disease or repeated heart attack? No one is sure. However, the wisest course would certainly seem to be the prudent course. "Eat, drink, and be merry" means eat and drink in such a way that you *can* be merry.

17

Take It Off

ARE YOU ONE of those people who thinks that you're not overweight, but that everyone else is undernourished? If so, take time now. Squeeze the skin folds over your stomach or sides, and see if there seems to be $1/2$ inch or more of tissue present. If there is, it's too much. Now look at the table on page 105. It shows the new svelte you that you could be.

Most adults in our society have a weight problem. After age 25, you end up gaining weight unless you do something about the food you eat and the amount of your daily activity. The reason is that, beginning at this age, your body starts to need less energy because your metabolism is slowing down. The result is that you require about 10 less calories every day for each year that passes, and if you don't cut back by this amount you'll end up gaining about a pound a year.

At age 26 you need 10 fewer calories than what you used to take in each day at age 25. And by age 35 your body's needs will have dropped 100 calories per day. Thus, a 45-year-old man who eats and exercises the same way he did 20 years ago will find himself weighing 20 pounds more. You don't have to eat a *lot* of extra food to become fat. People who stay thin

Your Ideal Weight
(Within 5- to 10-pound range)

HEIGHT (without shoes)	WEIGHT (WITHOUT CLOTHING)		
Men	Light build	Medium build	Heavy build
5 ft. 3 in.	118	129	141
5 ft. 4 in.	122	133	145
5 ft. 5 in.	126	137	149
5 ft. 6 in.	130	142	155
5 ft. 7 in.	134	147	161
5 ft. 8 in.	139	151	166
5 ft. 9 in.	143	155	170
5 ft. 10 in.	147	159	174
5 ft. 11 in.	150	163	178
6 ft.	154	167	183
6 ft. 1 in.	158	171	188
6 ft. 2 in.	162	175	192
6 ft. 3 in.	165	178	195
Women			
5 ft.	100	109	118
5 ft. 1 in.	104	112	121
5 ft. 2 in.	107	115	125
5 ft. 3 in.	110	118	128
5 ft. 4 in.	113	122	132
5 ft. 5 in.	116	125	135
5 ft. 6 in.	120	129	139
5 ft. 7 in.	123	132	142
5 ft. 8 in.	126	136	146
5 ft. 9 in.	130	140	151
5 ft. 10 in.	133	144	156
5 ft. 11 in.	137	148	161
6 ft.	141	152	166

Source: U.S. Department of Agriculture.

probably eat only about 3 percent less food than overweight people do.

Eating Can Be Hazardous to Your Health

Insurance company figures indicate that once you are 10 pounds over your ideal weight, each additional pound costs you a month of your life. In fact, to get an idea of what being overweight does to your health, consider the following figures:

For people who are overweight by:	The increase in the death rate is:
10%	13%
20%	25%
30%	40%

An overweight condition is also associated with an increased incidence of coronary artery disease, it often leads to high blood pressure, and it places a definite burden on the heart: the heart must work harder because every activity is more difficult for a heavy person.

The value of losing weight is tremendous:

- Hypertensive patients oftentimes have a significant improvement in their blood pressures.

- Blood fats—triglycerides—tend to return toward normal.

- Diabetics have less trouble handling sugar loads.

- Most important, you tend to feel better, feel less tired, and have a better self-image.

It's important to understand that virtually everyone can lose weight. Many people erroneously think the opposite, but being overweight seldom is due to familial or inherited factors or to "abnormal metabolism." Being overweight is simply the result of *bad habits*. It comes down to eating too much and being too inactive. After all, the best reducing exercise is placing both hands squarely against the table edge and pushing away.

Eating Well: Nourishing and Delicious Blends

In addition to watching your calories, you might as well start eating healthy foods. There are a number of nutritious ones, less fattening and low in cholesterol and saturated fats, and from all of these, you can begin to create some scrumptious delights.

- Fish

- Fruits and fruit juices, vegetables, nuts, seeds, sprouts, and crisp, tossed salads. (Fruits and vegetables also have a type of fiber that helps lower cholesterol, and foods with wheat and bran contain another fiber that may prevent cancer.)

- Nonfat dairy products and other low-calorie beverages

- Starches and pastas—should be a staple in every household

- Cereals and whole grains—the "whole" keeps the vitamins in

- Rice—simple white, rich brown, or bulgur wheat for that Middle Eastern flavor

- Peas, green beans, and other beans or "legumes," soy products; many of which are high in protein

- Combinations and flavors with garlic, onions, wine, glorious herbs, and mysterious spices—from around the world and from your own creativity

Tip the Scale Tips

How are you going to get those pounds off? There are literally hundreds of books written about dieting, and a great number of them aren't very good. While we do not plan to go into any of the programs, we will say this: There is no sense going on a crash diet every three months. It probably does more harm than good and evidence shows that you'll only put the weight back on. Diet pills aren't of any value either. There just aren't any temporary measures! You have to watch what you eat on a "continuing" basis and cut down on those calories . . . forever.

If you really want to take weight off or watch your weight, here are some ways to do it:

- Once you've made a commitment to lose weight, you need to set realistic goals—write them down and set up a workable timetable for achieving them.

- Since you've decided to lose weight, it's helpful to have a whole different *attitude* about your life. There are going to be tough moments, doubts, discouragements, impulses to give up, maybe even invitations to judge the local cake bake-off. This new attitude expects these adversities, knows they will pass, and that you're strong enough to withstand them and forge on.

- Keep a food diary. This helps you understand your eating habits; how you feel when you eat, whether you're hungry, tired, bored, unhappy. After looking this over, you will begin to see when and why you take in all those needless calories.

- Eat only when you are hungry. Learn to differentiate between true hunger and appetite. Hunger is an inborn instinct—your body needs food; whereas appetite is the *desire* for food and is usually a habit—one that can be changed.

- Listen to your body. If it's calling out for something sweet, that's okay in moderation. Most of the time your body is very sensible and will ask for a more balanced, nutritious diet.

- When you're eating, pay attention to the food. Chew and savor each morsel. Don't be distracted and find yourself off somewhere else, like in the middle of the TV soaps. Eat slowly and attentively, putting down your fork between each bite.

- Faced between meals with the urge to eat, drink, instead, a large glass of ice water.

- Exercise regularly. It probably takes only 30 to 45 minutes a day of exercise to counteract some of these excess calories you've taken in. You might want to try an aerobics class.

- Shop more carefully. Don't shop when you are hungry. You tend to buy everything you see.

- Cut down on the size of the portions you eat. Use smaller plates and bowls to make the portions look bigger and more appetizing. Arrange the food on the plate before bringing it to the table.

- Learn to leave some food on the plate. Stop eating when you feel comfortable and before you are full.

- Skip junk foods and those that add calories without offering many vitamins or minerals. For example—cocktails, fats, sugars and sugary foods such as canned fruits, soft drinks, sugar-coated breakfast cereals, honey, syrups, or rich desserts such as cakes and ice cream.

- Diet clinics may be very helpful if you can't go it alone. Be selective. Pick one that doesn't offer a lot of gimmicks or short-cut the principles we've laid out.

- Pretend there's more than one of you and you're having an imaginary conversation. Think—as you are planning to eat—Why are you eating right now? Will this food really satisfy your needs?

- Folks who are overweight often tend to focus on a negative self-image. Learn instead to focus on those parts of yourself that you love—that wonderful smile, those dimples, the way you sing off key.

- Keep visualizing to yourself how wonderful you're going to look when you're thin.

Of course, the key to all this is you have to *want* to control your weight. You have to be motivated. You have to want to break those bad eating habits. And in order to come to grips with those emotionally charged situations that lead to your eating or snacking, you must understand them and cope with them.

These are the general approaches. You can also count those calories more carefully. The table on the next page shows how many calories you should be taking in each day once you reach your ideal weight. Appendix F gives you the details of the calorie content of various foods, and Appendix G the calories expended in various physical activities.

Calorie Allowance for Adults
of Average Physical Activity

DESIRABLE WEIGHT	25 YEARS	45 YEARS	65 YEARS
Men			
110	2300	2050	1750
120	2400	2200	1850
130	2550	2300	1950
140	2700	2450	2050
150	2850	2550	2150
160	3000	2700	2250
170	3100	2800	2350
180	3250	2950	2450
190	3400	3050	2600
Women			
90	1600	1500	1250
100	1750	1600	1350
110	1900	1700	1450
120	2000	1800	1500
130	2100	1900	1600
140	2250	2050	1700
150	2350	2150	1800
160	2500	2250	1900

Source: U.S. Department of Agriculture.

Right now it may seem like an overwhelming undertaking to change that old body of yours. But thousands of people have learned to control their weight without much difficulty, simply because over the years they've knowingly or unknowingly developed many of the habits suggested above. Try some of them. Heads will turn when you walk in with that new wardrobe.

18

Drinking: One Martini,
Two Martini,
Three Martini, Four. . .

BET YOU'RE AFRAID we're going to tell you to stop drinking.
We're not.

By and large, alcohol is not a risk factor; it certainly does
not lead to coronary disease. (Some believe alcohol in moderation protects against coronary disease, perhaps by raising
HDL, but research on this is conflicting.) However, as long as
we're talking about putting things in your mouth, as we have
in the last two chapters, it is appropriate to talk about some
aspects of alcohol.

Alcohol isn't dangerous after a heart attack when it is consumed in moderation—that is, 2 to 3 ounces per day. It may
be necessary to restrict your intake, however, if you have a
high triglyceride level or a weight problem. In addition, you
should watch the drinking before and during exercise, since
alcohol dilates blood vessels, and this may result in your feeling faint while exercising.

Of course, excessive drinking and alcohol abuse is a serious
problem, not only in the United States but all over the world.
If you think you might be in this category of drinker, you
should be aware that excessive amounts of alcohol over long

periods of time may injure not only your liver but also your heart. For the average person who has angina pectoris or who has had a heart attack, however, one or two cocktails before dinner, or wine with dinner, or even an after-dinner drink can be enjoyed without risk. But four is more than more than enough.

19

Exercise: Lifting a Finger to Help Yourself

EVERYWHERE YOU TURN, people are out there exercising. And this is one fad that we think is "on the mark"—so let's get set and go with it.

How would you like your doctor to prescribe a pill that makes you:

- Less tired, anxious, and stressed

- Feel more confident

- Look more handsome and attractive

That's what exercise does. Exercise is probably one of the best "pills" for your overall health. So we don't agree with Erma Bombeck that the main reason to exercise is to hear deep breathing again.

Most experts aver that many years of an active life-style confers some protection from coronary fatality, and that exercising after a heart attack probably does the same, though no one is certain of this. In addition, an exercise program helps bring down the blood triglycerides when they're elevated and increases HDL which actually *protects* against the progress of coronary disease.

One thing, unfortunately, that exercise does *not* do: it does not stimulate the growth of new coronary arteries, of collateral vessels. Medical scientists had believed previously that it might do so, but this hasn't panned out in recent research.

But exercise, it has been philosophized, is the closest thing there is to an antiaging pill. And for heart patients in particular, exercise can help condition the heart so it works as efficiently as it is capable (indeed, some former heart patients have even become marathon runners—though we're not going to guarantee this in your case, or even suggest you try), as well as tone up other muscles, help you control your weight, control high blood pressure and diabetes, get back to work quicker, and help you return to a normal life.

And it need not be boring or threatening.

Of course you can't just put on sneakers and get out there. Perhaps more than any other area (except medication) this is where you have to work closely with your doctor.

Exercise Testing

First of all, he or she may ask you to take an exercise test or so-called *treadmill test* or stress EKG ("stress" doesn't mean worry here; it means effort on the heart). Exercise testing is used for many things. It is used to test people who haven't had heart attacks but have been inactive and want to start exercising again. It is used to diagnose coronary disease, to distinguish other conditions that might present similar symptoms, and to evaluate the severity of coronary disease. Finally, it's also used to follow the progress of patients who have had angioplasty or coronary bypass surgery. Many people do not need an exercise test; that's up to the physician.

In the treadmill test, you will have the same sort of electrocardiogram taken that we described earlier, only you will be required to have it done while walking or running on a motor-driven treadmill or while pedaling a stationary bicycle. Your heart needs to get more blood during exercise because it is working harder, and if it doesn't get up a sufficient blood

The treadmill exercise test

supply, certain changes often show up on the electrocardiogram. At the start of the test, the amount of exercise required is slight (a slow saunter), but as it continues, you will exercise more and more, perhaps reaching a run, reaching your peak. From this, the physician can see how well your heart responds to a work load by analyzing your electrocardiogram and the heart-rate and blood-pressure changes.

If you are having this test within the first 2 weeks after a heart attack, much less exercise will be required than 1 to 2 months later. You'll probably not even be asked to run but rather to walk somewhat briskly.

In addition, your doctor may want you to undergo the treadmill test using small quantities of a radioactive substance such as *thallium*. This is injected into your bloodstream in order to identify areas of the heart where the delivery of blood may be insufficient and to estimate the size of these areas. (Don't worry, this is a very low and safe amount of radioactivity, far less than those in x-rays, for example.)

So we use exercise testing to diagnose your condition, gauge its severity, and to determine the range of reasonable limits of exercise: too little may weaken you; too much might be dangerous. The test in effect helps your doctor design an exercise prescription for you to follow.

Easing into Exercise

It is terribly important that you start your exercise program *slowly*, despite the inclination to try and undo years of inactivity with an overzealous approach. Starting too vigorously is not only dangerous but will give you sore muscles and joints, which can only discourage you from further exercise. We are talking about *aerobic* exercise—the kind you do when you walk, jog, swim, or cycle.

One of the main goals during an exercise program is progressively to increase your heart rate. As we will see, you will be asked to achieve what are called *target heart rates*. During the early stages, while you are still in the hospital, the target heart rate that you initially reach will be up to only 100 or 110 beats per minute (for periods of 5 to 10 minutes at first). At home and as the months pass, your heart rate will be allowed to go to 120 to 130, then 130 to 150 beats per minute. Whatever your rate of progress, the program will be individually tailored for you.

The way to monitor your heart rate is to take your pulse. You should learn to do this yourself, so that you can tell when you have reached your reasonable limits of physical activity. Taking a pulse is easy and can be learned from your doctor or nurse in a few minutes. A pulse can be taken on a wrist (with index and middle finger), on the neck, or (if you're not shy) in the groin. You'll need a watch with a second hand. Count the number of pulses that occur in a half minute, and multiply by 2 to get your heartbeats per minute (or beats in 10 seconds multiplied by 6).

Taking your pulse

Exercise Tips

As we noted in Chapter 2, you will already have started exercising in the hospital, with the help of a nurse or physical therapist. Here we are concerned about easing you into exercise after you get home.

SOME DON'TS:

• Don't strain against or lift extremely heavy objects.

• Don't do sudden or rapid activity, such as fast running.

• On the other hand, don't do stationary exercise (isometric exercise), in which the muscles are tightly flexed but there is no movement.

• Don't exercise if you feel unusually fatigued or ill.

• Don't take hot or cold showers or baths before and after exercise. They may lead to a fall in blood pressure or irregular heartbeat. (Moderately warm water is O.K.)

• Don't drink alcohol for an hour before and after exercise.

• Don't get into heavy competitive games.

SOME DO'S:

• *Warm up* for 5 to 10 minutes before the exercise session with light calisthenics, including stretching, twisting, touching toes, bending at the waist, bending knees and elbows, or otherwise moving the limbs (but avoid straining). Warming up not only limbers you and so prevents bone, muscle, and joint injuries; it also protects your heart against unnecessary stress, since you are beginning gradually.

• Do start exercising on level ground, avoiding hills. It's a good idea to begin any jogging on a soft surface such as a cinder track to avoid the injuries that can occur when running on a hard street or sidewalk. Once you get used to exercise, you can move on to these harder surfaces. Proper running or walking shoes are a must to prevent musculo-skeletal injuries.

Warm up

Exercise

Cool down

- Do *cool down* for 3 to 5 minutes after exercise, gradually diminishing but not stopping the exercise. This prevents large amounts of blood from "pooling" in the legs, which can cause dizziness and even fainting.

- Do ask your doctor about exercising at (or traveling to) places at high altitudes. Most heart-attack patients can tolerate elevations between 3,500 and 6,000 feet well, but some people are troubled by angina or shortness of breath over 7,000 feet. In any event, remember that any type of exercise takes more energy at these higher elevations, so you should exercise less than you normally do, especially the first day or so while you're becoming acclimatized. Good physical conditioning several weeks before can minimize the effects of high altitude. Don't hesitate to take a nap if you're tired and remember the effects of alcohol, tranquilizers, and sedatives can be heightened at high altitudes.

Danger Zone

Be aware of the following *danger signs* while you are exercising. If any of them happen, consult your doctor.

- Severe or unusual fatigue.

- Dizziness or fainting during or after exercise.

- Unusually heavy perspiration.

- Irregular or unusually rapid heartbeat.

- Unusual shortness of breath (especially if it prevents you from speaking after you have stopped the exercise).

- Your heart rate does not return to normal within 10 minutes after exercise is over.

- New chest pain or pain that remains after you stop. (If you're taking nitroglycerin tablets, and 3 or 4 tablets and 15 minutes of rest do not make the pain go away, see your physician immediately.)

How Much Exercise Do You Need?

Scientists often divide this into four categories: frequency, intensity, duration, and type.

FREQUENCY: 3 to 5 times per week

INTENSITY: 60 to 90 percent of your maximum heart rate. You may want to ask your doctor or an exercise expert exactly what the intensity of your exercise should be.

DURATION: 20 to 60 minutes

TYPE: Aerobic

Aerobic exercise, such as walking, jogging, swimming, or cycling, is a type of exercise in which you breathe in enough oxygen to keep up with the requirements of your muscles. (This, by the way, contrasts with anaerobic exercise, a type of exercise such as isometrics, weightlifting, or sprinting, in which you don't take in sufficient oxygen to meet the needs of the muscles.)

Although aerobic exercise is the principal key to cardiovascular fitness, a certain amount of "strengthening exercise" may be supplemented if you wish. Strengthening exercise, including the use of weightlifting machines, tones up the muscles, shapes the body, makes you appear more aesthetically pleasing, and you end up feeling less tired. Although weight training does not specifically condition the cardiovascular system, it does strengthen the muscles you use in aerobic exercise, which in turn improves your aerobic capacity.

High-Impact vs. Low-Impact Aerobics

Jogging and running, among the best of the aerobic exercises, suffer from one tremendous liability—that being they pound your muscles, bones, and joints and lead to innumerable injuries. Therefore, these are termed *high-impact* aerobic exercises.

More and more, then, people are turning to *low-impact* aerobic exercises, among the best of which are swimming, cycling, and some forms of aerobic dance. Walking, in fact, is an excellent form of low-impact aerobic exercise, but you have to give it at least an hour each day since it is a much lower "intensity" exercise. Remember, you can condition your cardiovascular system even with walking!

After a while you may want to try two or three different types of exercise in order to: (1) condition more of your muscles; (2) keep down the amount of high-impact exercise; (3) avoid boredom and make exercise more enjoyable; (4) adapt more readily to change in weather or season. The better rounded your exercise program is, the easier it is to adapt to any activities in life, whether they be raising a barn, climbing a hill, tossing a football to one of your kids, or rushing through the usual work day.

Injuries

If you do suffer a minor injury while exercising, recite the magic incantation "rice."

R—Rest the injured area. You don't have to stop exercising entirely.

I—Ice, immediately and for the first 1 to 2 days.

C—Compression, some form of elastic bandage.

E—Elevation of the injured part.

Your Exercise Program

As we stated, your precise exercise program will be worked out between you and your doctor or physical therapist. Remember, though, that the two things to watch for are:

- *Your target heart rate*—which you monitor by taking your pulse. The aim of all exercise programs is to *gradually* increase the work load on the heart—that is, gradually over a period of time, increase the target heart rate.

- *Potential danger*—excessive fatigue, chest pain, shortness of breath, irregular heart rate.

On the next three pages are three exercise programs that your doctor may prescribe or modify. If they seem boring or threatening, talk it out with him or her. Perhaps some modifications can be made. Remember that a good exercise program gradually *increases the degree and duration of activity* over a period of days, weeks, and months.

PROGRAM #1: LIGHT CONDITIONING.   This is for the first 2 to 8 weeks following a heart attack, and involves leisurely and then more brisk *walking*. Some persons, particularly the elderly, may not want to proceed beyond this program. You start by walking leisurely for 10 to 20 minutes, and by the third or fourth week for longer periods of 30 to 40 minutes.

After the fourth week, the exercise is divided into segments of 5-minute periods of leisurely walking and 5-minute periods of slightly more brisk walking, in which you try to achieve target heart rates of 110 to 115 beats per minute during the brisker periods. This is done at first for 30 to 40 minutes, and by the fifth to sixth weeks, for 40 to 50 minutes.

Finally, between the sixth and eighth weeks, you should be walking the entire 45- to 50-minute periods at a brisk pace, maintaining the target heart rate of 110 to 115 beats per minute. The approximate distances during each of these stages are shown in the table on the following page.

PROGRAM #2: ACTIVE CONDITIONING.   Begun 8 weeks after a heart attack, this program combines walking and jogging 30 to 45 minutes three or more times a week. You begin by *jogging* 30 paces and *walking* 60 paces, continuing for about 30 minutes, during which you achieve a target heart rate of approximately 130 beats per minute while jogging, slowing down to 110 beats per minute or less while walking. As the months go by, the duration of exercise is lengthened, as the amount of jogging is increased and the period that you walk is decreased. At the same time, the target heart rate goes up, so that, for example, at $2^{1}/_{2}$ to 4 months, a target heart rate of 130 to 150 is reached while jogging, slowing to 130 or below while walking. After the first six months, jogging occupies the entire exercise period, reaching target rates of 135 to 155, the exercise periods lasting 30 to 45 minutes.

Exercise Program #1: Light Conditioning

TIME AFTER HEART ATTACK (WEEKS)	TYPE OF EXERCISE	DURATION OF EXERCISE (MINUTES)	APPROXIMATE DISTANCE (MILES)
2–3	Leisurely walk	15–20	½–¾
3–4	Leisurely walk	30–40	¾–1¼
4–5	Alternate 5 min. each leisurely and brisk walking. Target heart rates: under 110 (leisurely), 110–115 (brisk)	30–40	1¼–1½
5–6	Alternate 5 min. each leisurely and brisk walking. Target heart rates: under 110 (leisurely) 110–115 (brisk)	40–50	1½–2
6–8	Brisk walking only. Target heart rates: 110–115	45–50	2½–4
8	Begin Exercise Program #2, or continue with 6–8 week program.		

Exercise Program #2: Active Conditioning

TIME AFTER HEART ATTACK (MONTHS)	PACES WALKED	HEART RATE	PACES JOGGED	TARGET HEART RATE	TOTAL DURATION (MINUTES)
2–2¼	60	110	30	130	30
2¼–2½	30	110	30	130	30
2½–3	60	120	60	130	30
3–4	60	120	90	150	30–40
4–5	60	130	120	150	30–40
5–6	60	130	180	150	30–40
Over 6			All jogged	155	30–45

PROGRAM #3: ALTERNATIVE ACTIVE CONDITIONING. If you find walking and jogging too boring, this program, which also begins 8 weeks after a heart attack, permits swimming or riding a regular or stationary bicycle, if your doctor approves.

Exercise Program #3: Alternative Active Conditioning

TIME AFTER HEART ATTACK (MONTHS)	DURATION OF SLOW EXERCISE (MINUTES)	DURATION OF BRISK EXERCISE (MINUTES)	TARGET HEART RATE (FOR BRISK EXERCISE)	TOTAL DURATION (MINUTES)
2–2½	1	½	130	30
2½–3	1	1	130	30
3–4	1	1½	150	30–40
4–5	1	2	150	30–40
5–6	1	3	150	30–40
Over 6	1	3	155	30–40

Remember, these exercise programs are only examples. Some of you, especially if you are elderly or have bone or joint problems, may have difficulty reaching a high heart rate, but we now know that you can still condition your heart by exercising less vigorously but longer—say 30 to 60 minutes.

And if you take beta or calcium blocking medicines, the target heart rate set by your doctor may well be below 150.

Other Activities

As your heart gets stronger and you develop more endurance, you may want to switch to other kinds of activity—again, if your physician approves. One way to evaluate other forms of activity is to see what their energy cost is. These are expressed as *MET values,* which have nothing to do with baseball but are multiples of the amount of energy that you are using while just resting. The MET values of different kinds of activities are given in Appendix H.

If you plan to take up activities that are going to require more than a minimal amount of strain on your *arms,* you may also want to begin exercising them. At first try simple calisthenics, the flexing and stretching exercises we discussed. Then, over the next few weeks, practice lifting light objects, such as canned goods, raising them above your head and out to the side or in front of you with your arms extended. Start by lifting them five times; as you get stronger, you may lift them 10, 15, and eventually 20 times.

For exercise to do its job, you must do it at least three times a week. Make sure, therefore, that it isn't boring or threatening. Make sure it's fun.

20

Take Your Medicine

AMERICANS HAVE TAKEN so many over-the-counter and pre-scription drugs over the years that they have become accus-tomed to them as part of their daily lives. As a result, they frequently fail to respect fully the danger of using potent drugs or medications, which have the potential for doing harm as well as good unless they are used properly.

Your Medication Guide

Here are ten simple but important tips to make sure your medicines work for you and not against you.

- *Learn the names of the medications you are taking and do your best to understand why you are taking them.* That doesn't mean that you should second-guess your physician or try to acquire an instant medical education. It does mean, however, that you should be as informed as possible about what you are putting into your body.

- *Take medications in the amounts and at the times ordered by your physician.* Some patients have a tendency to modify the

127

dosage of medications prescribed, which can have serious consequences. Your body normally is an orderly and highly complex chemistry laboratory, and an improper dosage of some drugs can lead to certain physical changes you may find difficult to tolerate. Taking more medication than the amount your physician ordered may not only be less effective, it may be dangerous. Skipping doses can be equally bad. It is particularly hazardous when you attempt to catch up with missed doses by doubling up on future doses. Certain drugs should be taken before, with, or after meals. Remember that, most of the time, *you* are the most essential element in the treatment, because *you* administer the remedy.

- *Don't stop taking a medication that has been prescribed for you without first consulting your physician about it.* Some drugs are most effective only when the series of dosage is completed. Others may do more harm than good if they are stopped prematurely or suddenly. Don't fall into the subtle trap of stopping "by accident" because your supply ran out and you failed to have it refilled.

- *Check with your physician before taking any medications, whether prescribed or not.* Certain drugs interact with one another. The result can be that they interfere with each other or increase the reaction you may have to each of them. The consequences may be far different from what you anticipated. Even over-the-counter drug preparations such as aspirin and cold remedies contain chemicals that sometimes can be harmful when taken under some conditions, and they may react adversely with prescription medications you are taking.

- *Don't take medications prescribed for someone else.* A physician prescribes *individually,* for the unique conditions found in *each* patient. Since we're all different, each of us may react differently to the same medication.

- *Be sure to contact your physician if you have any reaction to a medication you did not anticipate.* Every drug has a large number of possible side effects—and they may be some you can't tolerate.

- *Keep all medications out of the reach of small children.* Some children are attracted to the bright colors or the smell and taste. They also often imitate what they see adults do, and will try to take your medicine.

- *Don't take medicines that have expired or are more than a couple of years old.* And flush down the toilet any drugs you are disposing of. Don't put them in a wastebasket for someone else to take.

- *Keep each medicine in its own labeled container.* Under no circumstances should a number of different pills be tossed together in one bottle.

- *Bring all of your medications with you when you visit your physician.* It is usually the best way to identify what you have been taking. Many pills are the same shape and color, and that similarity may make it difficult for you to describe accurately the prescriptions that you have at home.

Side Effects

Any drug has the potential for causing a wide range of unwanted side effects. Aspirin, for instance, is responsible for more than 20 of them.

Side effects to various drugs may include:

- Allergic reactions—fever, rash, itching, aching joints, yellow skin, swelling of hands or face, or difficult breathing

- Nausea, vomiting, or diarrhea

- Fatigue

- Falling blood count

Some side effects are mild and can be ignored. Some are disturbing and cause discomfort but usually can be controlled or relieved by a change in dosage of the medication taken or a change of the medication itself. Other side effects are potentially dangerous, requiring that your physician be notified. Some of the more common side effects to cardiovascular drugs are given in Appendix A.

Name that Pill

If your medicines are very costly, you might want to shop around, buy in quantity, and ask your doctor if he or she can prescribe generic drugs. While you are still in the hospital, your physician, nurse, or other member of the health recovery team will tell you:

- The name of the medication you are taking.
- How to tell it apart from other medications.
- The reason your physician prescribed it.
- Some of its side effects.
- Any special precautions you should use.

As you prepare for discharge from the hospital, you will again be instructed in the identifying characteristics (such as color, size, and shape) and use of the drugs prescribed for you. You may decide to keep a drug calendar such as the one on the opposite page. A number of gadgets are available in your drugstore to help you keep track of your medications. Read Appendix A for more details about these medications. It is essential to your recovery and comfort that you understand everything you can about them.

	MON		TUE		WED		THUR		FRI		SAT		SUN	
	AM	PM	AM	PM	AM	PM	AM	PM	AM	PM	AM	PM	AM	PM
Drug: Digoxin	8		8		8		8		8		8		8	
Amount: 0.25 mg./pill														
Dosage: I pill each day														
Drug: Hydrochlorothiazide	8	5	8	5	8	5	8	5	8	5	8	5	8	5
Amount: 50 mg./pill														
Dosage: I pill twice a day														
Drug: Potassium Chloride	8	5	8	5	8	5	8	5	8	5	8	5	8	5
Amount: 20 mEq. / I tsp.														
Dosage: I tsp twice a day														
Drug: Coumadin	8				8				8				8	
Amount: 5 mg./pill														
Dosage: I pill every other day														

Drug calendar

21

Your Sex Life

DO YOU HAVE TO stop having sex? Of course not, you sexy creature. In fact, it is *desirable* to resume your usual sex life: mutually loving relationships are extremely important, and particularly so following a heart attack.

Isn't there some danger? Not particularly. Sex is, after all, a form of mild to moderate physical activity. The stress on the cardiovascular system and increased blood pressure, heart rate, and respiration rate during sex is no more than that of climbing a couple of flights of stairs. While some people may suffer a bit of anginal chest pain during sex, it is usually rapidly alleviated with immediate rest and, occasionally, a nitroglycerin tablet. You simply should not be timid about going back to your usual sex life.

As you might expect, the most frequent question patients ask about sex is: When can I resume? This is up to your physician, who knows how severe your heart injury was. You should not begin an active sex life without first discussing it with your doctor. In most cases, however, sex can be resumed in 3 to 6 weeks after the heart attack.

The Joy of Sex

Here are some suggestions that help you resume a satisfying sex life:

- A loving and considerate act of love should take place in a calm and serene atmosphere. Avoid arguments or emotional discussions that cause you or your partner unnecessary excitement or anxiety. If there were any unresolved tensions associated with sex before your heart attack, they will probably continue to be a problem, and you should not feel reluctant about seeking psychological counseling. Either partner may become fearful of having sex—fear either of the activity itself or the accompanying excitement. These emotions are often needlessly exaggerated. Open communication between the two of you goes a long way toward dealing with these anxieties.

- Find positions comfortable for both of you. Sex need not involve gymnastics to be satisfying. You should have no hesitancy about following sexual preferences that you and your partner find mutually comfortable.

- Avoid having sex when you are unduly fatigued.

- Avoid having sex immediately after eating a meal, since the digestive system will be making heavy demands on the blood supply, and the additional demand required during sexual activity may place the heart under unusual strain.

- Avoid sex in locations where it is very hot or very cold, since your cardiovascular system will already be under the stress of controlling your body's temperature.

- Avoid drinking a lot of alcohol before sex. A small amount may help relax you, but large amounts will dilate the blood vessels, causing an increase in the heart rate, which means the heart has to work harder.

- If you've lost interest or developed any sexual problems, it may be because you're depressed or frightened. This is not at all uncommon. It happens to others and in all likelihood is transitory. Time and mutual understanding are generally all that's necessary. However you may decide that counseling would be beneficial.

- Some drugs such as tranquilizers, beta blockers, or those used to control high blood pressure may interfere with sexual performance. If they do, call your physician. An adjustment in the amount, type, or time of taking the medication may be all that is required.

Sex is, of course, a form of physical exercise. Thus, the better your physical fitness and muscle tone, the less strain on your cardiovascular system.

Caveats

If you sometimes feel anginal chest pain during sex, here's what to do:

- Take one or two nitroglycerin tablets *before* you begin to become aroused.
- Take nitroglycerin tablets to relieve chest pain developing during the sexual activity. Don't take more than a total of three over a short period of time. (If you need more, that means you need to see a physician.)
- Rest for 15 to 30 minutes before resuming sexual activity.

You should seek medical attention when:

- The angina pain remains unrelieved after you've taken three or more nitroglycerin tablets.
- Rest and inactivity do not relieve the pain.
- You feel a higher than normal heartbeat or irregular heart rhythm.
- Sweating lasts more than 15 minutes after orgasm.

Don't let this list of cautions deter you from beginning to reactivate your sex life. We all need love, in sickness and in health—and that includes you and your partner.

22

Going Back to Work

ONE OF THE MOST frequently asked questions we hear is, "When can I go back to work?" You will be happy to learn that about 85 percent of patients with uncomplicated myocardial infarctions sooner or later return to work.

Most return within the first 6 weeks to 3 months, but it is not unusual to take longer. Just when you go back is a decision to be worked out between you and your doctor. Here are some of the factors that will enter into the decision:

- The severity of your heart attack and how much heart muscle is damaged.

- The speed of your recovery. Although, as might be expected, older people take longer to bounce back than younger ones, recovery is still an individual matter. A lot depends, of course, on what kind of shape you were in before the heart attack.

- How hard you work to make yourself healthy again— whether you lose weight, get to exercising, and so on.

- The kind of job you hold—for example, desk work versus heavy-labor job.

137

Simulation

After 3 to 6 weeks as your recovery proceeds, it's a good idea to *simulate* your work activity at home. If you have a desk job involving lots of decisions and interruptions and phone calls, set up a situation with a co-worker in which you are called with questions from time to time throughout the day (start this gradually, of course—we don't want you tense about day-to-day problems on the job when you're only just out of the hospital). If you're in more of a manufacturing or laboring occupation, see if you can set up some shop or gardening activity that approximates what you do. (Or, under the watchful eye of your doctor, you might get a treadmill test.) The idea of all this is to see whether the work is going to bother you.

Some types of jobs permit employees to go back part time. If this is so in your field, by all means do it this way. If you cannot, then don't try to jump the gun—wait until your physician says it's O.K.

In some cases, where the job is an unusually strenuous one, or if you remain very ill, it may be best to face the facts and consider changing jobs—or even changing occupations. Look under "Vocational Consultants" in the Yellow Pages of the phone book, or call your city or county social services department for a recommendation on a vocational counselor, if it seems like this might be the best choice for you. Discuss it with your doctor.

Money

The real question behind the question as to when one can return to work is, in most cases, a question about money. Few of us feel we can go without working for long because few of us have the wherewithal to go a long time without income and not have a reduced standard of living.

If you feel this might be the case, don't sit around worrying about it. Get some advice. Get your spouse or a friend researching your job benefits. Have someone look into worker's compensation. See what insurance policies apply. If you have an accountant or a lawyer, take up the matter with him or her. Don't let yourself get into an emotional funk about it.

Driving

As a footnote to the subject of returning to work, we should say something about driving. When will you be able to resume driving a car again? This is a tricky question that can only be answered by your physician. Most driving is not taxing and can be resumed in 2 to 4 weeks. However, in heavy traffic, driving can produce increased heart rates, and your doctor may advise you to wait a while before undertaking this kind of driving again. Some states require a physician's approval before a person can return to driving after a heart attack.

The main point to keep in mind is that most people return to productive employment after their heart attack and are able to continue working for years to come. Who was it who said that among his great loves was "love of work"?

23

Recovery for Older People

IF IT SOMEHOW SEEMS like we've been talking to the under-65s in this book (as in the preceding chapter on going back to work), we do not mean that to be the case. The book is for everyone.

Now, it is true that people age in different ways, and many people in their seventies and over are "younger"—more alive, alert, and active–than people half their age, and so are apt to recover from a heart attack as effectively as any younger person. Even so, there are some special considerations to be aware of if you or someone you know is a heart patient over 70.

The Recovery Period

Because in older people many things heal more slowly (even a cut finger) and because the heart has less overall reserve capacity, and thus is somewhat less able to withstand the damage caused by a heart attack, the recovery period consequently may be longer—perhaps several weeks or months longer. In addition, many elderly people may suffer from a variety of other illnesses present before the attack, and these too may affect recovery time.

Yet, at the same time, there is probably less need to return to a highly active life. Few people in their late seventies work at a full-time job. Many at that age are happy to spend their time with their retirement interests and with their family and friends.

After the patient has left the hospital and is recuperating at home, it's generally a good idea to be sure he or she is not left alone or not left alone with a spouse or friend who is also ill.

Some older people may have vision problems, so that they find it difficult to read medication and other instructions, or they may have failings of memory so that they forget to take their medicines.

To help with medical problems and with the general running of the household, the patient should be provided with care by family members, live-in help, or members of the local visiting nurses' association. Family members in particular should learn as much as they can about heart attacks and coronary disease.

Therapy

Because some elderly people tend to be less flexible, less able to change time-worn habits, family members and physicians are advised to take a less-rigid line and settle for compromises rather than insist the patient follow every instruction exactly. Though medications should be taken *precisely* as prescribed, everything else we have discussed in this book—diet modifications, exercise programs, even stopping smoking—are less important. (However, if severe high blood pressure or congestive heart failure are present, it may be important to follow a low-salt diet.)

Of course, the patient should be encouraged to be as active as possible, but a structured exercise program may not be possible, especially if the patient is confined to bed. And given the dangers of falling and fracturing a bone, it may not even be desirable. However, every elderly patient, to the extent possible, should be encouraged to get up and move about to some degree.

Medication can pose a problem, not only because elderly patients may have vision and memory difficulties, but also because they seem to be somewhat less tolerant of medications and are more likely to develop undesirable side effects. For example, nitroglycerin may produce a marked fall in blood pressure in older people and so should be administered very carefully. After taking nitroglycerin, an elderly person should not stand up suddenly within the first 5 minutes.

Digitalis may also produce more undesirable reactions in older persons, and a patient and his or her family should be very aware of the potential side effects (see Chapter 20 and Appendix A), so that the warning signs will be recognized should they appear.

Although it is true that recovery may not rejuvenate an older coronary patient, this does not mean that one cannot come back to a happy, active, productive life. You, like red wine, can age well.

24

Heart Clubs

THIS MAY BE the shortest chapter in the book, but it's an important one. Its message is: You are not alone. As we stated earlier, nearly a million and a half people suffer heart attacks every year.

Many of these people have gotten together in heart clubs or support groups organized either by health professionals or by patients themselves. Just as groups of people like yourself can often help you in quitting smoking or losing weight, so other heart patients can help you in understanding what you should or should not do, assist you in starting an exercise program and retooling your eating habits, and answering questions you have. Thus, when we're asked whether it's worth looking into heart clubs, our answer is: Yes. In spades.

Ask the staff at your hospital about them. Or call your local heart association.

25

Coronary Angiography and
Coronary Angioplasty

LET'S LOOK AT *high-tech* cardiology for a moment.

Coronary Angiography

When a special x-ray picture of your coronary arteries is
needed, your physician may recommend a coronary angiogram. This test involves the injection of a special dye into the
coronary arteries. The dye can be seen on x-ray film as it
flows through the arteries, and thus any obstruction of the
coronary arteries can be seen and the location and severity of
narrowing can be pinpointed.

The test is usually done in the hospital. An area of the groin
or arm is numbed with a local anesthetic (such as novocaine).
One of the blood vessels passing through the arm or groin is
entered by a needle or tiny incision, and a thin, long tube (a
catheter) is passed through this vessel to an area just outside
the heart, where its tip is directed into the openings of the
coronary arteries. Then the dye is injected into the arteries,
x-ray movies or still shots are taken, and the films are analyzed
to locate regions of narrowing within the coronary arteries.

Coronary Angioplasty: Balloon Dilatation

One of the more exciting and new forms of treatment for coronary artery narrowing is coronary angioplasty. This therapy begins very much like coronary angiography. A tube with a small deflated balloon at its tip is inserted through the groin or arm and threaded to the heart. The tube is guided into the area where the coronary artery is obstructed and the balloon is inflated, compressing the obstructing fatty plaque against the artery wall and widening the passageway so that more blood can reach the heart muscle.

Certainly this treatment isn't needed routinely, and the decision whether or not it would be best for you depends on a host of facts, such as your particular symptoms, which of the arteries are obstructed, and what kind of heart attack you had. Sometimes angioplasty is used in the first hours of a heart attack, or, at times, days or weeks later. Or alternatively, it's been used in people with angina who have not suffered a heart attack.

Angioplasty is remarkably effective, and upward of 9 out of 10 people in whom it is tried are initially improved, though sometimes an area of narrowing recurs and the artery has to be reopened a second time.

This novel procedure has a great deal going for it—it's simple, it's fairly safe, and, most encouragingly, it works! After all, we've been looking for something like a Roto-Rooter for years, and this is the closest we've come.

26

Coronary Bypass Surgery

IT IS AMAZING the number of people who have had heart and coronary problems who ask us about the subject of bypass surgery—even though for most there is little chance they would be candidates for it. Nevertheless, it is an important and fascinating subject, so let's describe it here.

In some cases, the best way to keep an adequate supply of blood flowing into the heart is to surgically implant more blood vessels to act as additional coronary arteries. This procedure is called *coronary bypass surgery* or *aortocoronary (AC) bypass surgery.*

Most patients with angina pectoris or who have suffered heart attacks can be treated perfectly well without this operation. However, it is recommended for patients with worsening or severe angina that does not improve with standard medication and for some patients with very severe coronary disease, particularly some with obstruction of three major vessels or with obstruction of the left main coronary artery.

The first bypass operation was performed in 1964, and by now upward of 100,000 procedures per year are performed in the United States. It is a relatively safe procedure, with a 90 to 95 percent or greater chance of one's getting through the operation. If disabling angina is present, there is a high likelihood that the pain will be diminished or eliminated. The

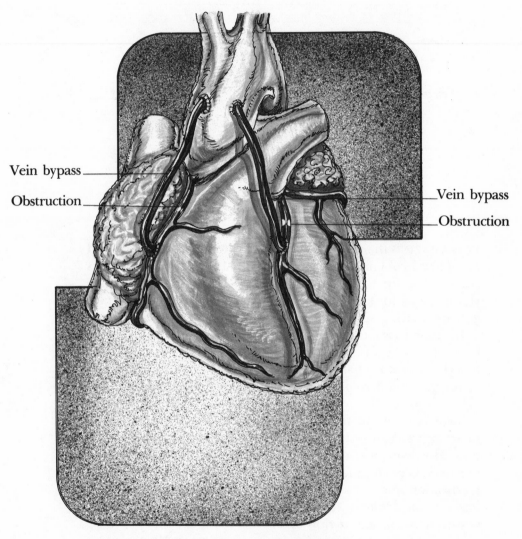

Vein bypass

Obstruction

Vein bypass

Obstruction

Coronary artery bypass

surgery also prolongs lives of some patients with narrowing of particularly critical areas of the coronary system.

However, despite such gratifying results, the procedure will not *necessarily* eliminate angina pain in all patients or prevent heart attacks from occurring, and will not delay the progression of atherosclerosis. Even after 20 years of experience, there is still a great deal to be learned about the results of such operations.

The decision as to whether you should have bypass surgery should never be made lightly. A number of questions should be considered by you, your family, and physician together, among them:

- How old are you?
- How able are you to work or live the kind of life you desire?
- How incapacitating is the angina?
- Are symptoms progressive?
- How well do you respond to medications?
- What are the results of your exercise tests?
- What is the severity of coronary narrowing?

In addition to these factors, you and your doctor must weigh the potential *benefits* of the operation against the *risks* of surgery. Don't be hustled into surgery. If you have any doubts, get more facts from your physician, or if you feel the need, you can always get a second opinion.

How the Bypass Operation Is Done

If it is decided to proceed with bypass surgery, the patient is put to sleep with a general anesthetic. While the operation is in progress, a life-support system called a *heart-lung machine* is connected to the patient's circulatory system, to temporarily relieve the heart and lungs of their normal function while the heart is being worked on. This is called *open-heart surgery*, and it is used in other cardiac conditions such as replacement or repair of diseased valves or correction of congenital birth defects such as holes in the heart.

The operation is accomplished by taking a piece of vein from the patient's leg (occasionally an artery from the inner chest is used, the internal mammary artery) and securing it from the aorta to a portion of coronary artery beyond the point of obstruction. This way, it is used to *bypass* (detour) blood around the area of the blocked artery.

Other Operations in Coronary Disease

After some serious heart attacks, a pouch or bulge forms on the left ventricular muscle called a *ventricular aneurysm.* Most of these produce no problems, but if they are very large, they can cause congestive failure or rhythm disturbances. In such instances, it may be necessary to surgically excise the aneurysm—a procedure called *ventricular aneurysmectomy.*

In other cases, the mitral valve may develop a leak after a heart attack. Most of the time the leak is very slight and produces no problems whatever, but in rare cases an excessive amount of blood may leak through the valve, congestive failure may develop, and the valve may need to be replaced surgically.

There are now a great number of artificial (prosthetic) valves available for replacement. Some are made out of cloth, metal, and plastic (the so-called *mechanical ball or disc valves,* for example) and some are actually made partly from the heart valves of pigs. These tissue valves are "cured"—meaning they are not alive—and therefore aren't rejected, as may happen in heart transplantation. The tissue valves are mounted on a cloth-covered ring that can be sewn in place.

When performed on carefully selected patients, bypass grafting and the other operations are extremely useful therapy. However, again it must be stressed that most people with heart attacks or angina do admirably well without surgery.

27

A Salvage Job

OCCASIONALLY DURING the *early* throes of a heart attack your doctor may try a "salvage job." The plan here is to try to preserve and keep alive areas of heart muscle that are endangered with or undergoing a myocardial infarction by opening or bypassing a coronary artery that has become blocked.

Among the more modern approaches to heart attack, "salvaging" is by no means to be tried in all cases. In fact, medical scientists are just beginning to wrestle with when it should and should not be considered.

Three techniques for salvaging areas of heart muscle which are in danger are: (1) reopening the obstructed artery with balloon coronary angioplasty—done hours, days, or even weeks after the heart attack; (2) coronary bypass surgery—the detour operation; and (3) by injecting a medicine that will open the closed coronary passageway—a technique known as *thrombolysis* (dissolving the thrombus or clot, the mass that is producing the obstruction).

Certain kinds of heart attack develop when a part of the coronary vessel suddenly becomes stopped up, when the blood clots (sort of gels) within the artery and blood flow ceases—very much like a logjam in a river. If the clot can be caught soon—the earlier the better, preferably within the first 3 to 4 hours—it can be dissolved, yet another reason to get to the hospital quickly if an attack is suspected. The clot is dissolved by injecting medicine either into the vein or directly into the coronary artery (during coronary angiography). Streptokinase, urokinase, and TPA (initials for a very fancy-named medicine, tissue plasminogen activator) are three medications used for such purposes, TPA being the newest and safest of the three. Sometimes the injected medicine only partly opens the artery, and later more blood can be brought to the heart by employing an angioplasty or bypass operation.

As mentioned, we are just beginning to explore this new high-tech approach, and no one is yet sure just when it should be tried or how successful it's going to turn out to be. But what we do know so far is that it is possible *some of the time* to limit the size of the damage, to get the heart to beat a little more vigorously, and, perhaps, to get through the heart attack more safely. And you have to admit, this sounds intriguing.

The Days Ahead

WE COULD HAVE called this book *Ten Easy Steps to Recovering from Your Heart Attack* and retired on the royalties.

But the title would not be honest. There are no easy steps to coming back. Yet the experience of millions shows that it is possible, and we're sure it's possible for you.

Now you know the basics. What follows—the glossary and the detailed appendixes—are intended as further explorations. There's a lot you can do—not just to recover but to expand the quality of your life.

This is not the end. It is the beginning.

Glossary

ACUTE (*ah-CUTE*) Indicates illness that appears suddenly or is of short duration.

AEROBIC EXERCISE (*air-ROBE-ic*) An endurance type of exercise, such as walking, jogging, swimming, or cycling, used to increase overall, and particularly cardiovascular, fitness.

ANGINA PECTORIS (*AN-jin-ah PEC-tor-us*) Chest discomfort or pain due to a temporary inadequacy of blood to an area of heart muscle.

ANGIOCARDIOGRAPHY (*AN-jee-oh-kar-dee-OG-rah-fee*) An x-ray examination of the heart or arteries. Performed by injecting a special dye into the bloodstream, so that the inside of the heart and blood vessels can be seen on either still or moving x-ray film. *See also* Coronary angiography.

ANGIOGRAM (*AN-jee-oh-gram*) The x-ray picture obtained from angiography or angiocardiography.

ANGIOGRAPHY (*an-jee-OG-rah-fee*) X-ray examinations of areas of the body, performed by injecting special dyes. *See* Angiocardiography.

ANGIOPLASTY (*AN-gee-oh-plas-tee*) A technique for unblocking coronary obstruction by inflating a balloon which is

157

attached to a catheter and squeezing and thereby compressing the obstructing plaque.

ANOXIA (*an-OKS-see-ah*) Lack or deficiency of oxygen.

ANTERIOR DESCENDING CORONARY ARTERY The coronary artery that supplies blood to the front wall of the heart. Also called Left Anterior Descending or LAD. *See* Coronary artery.

ANTICOAGULANT (*ant-eye-koh-AG-u-lant*) Drug that delays blood clotting.

ANTIHYPERTENSIVE AGENT (*ant-eye-high-per-TEN-siv A-gent*) Drug that lowers blood pressure.

AORTA (*ay-OR-tah*) Main artery carrying blood from the principal pumping chamber of the heart, the left ventricle, to the other arteries and then to all parts of the body.

AORTIC INSUFFICIENCY (*ay-OR-tik in-suh-FISH-en-see*) Improper closing of the valve between the aorta and the lower left chamber of the heart, the left ventricle, thereby permitting a back-flow of blood into the ventricle.

AORTIC STENOSIS (*ay-OR-tik ste-NOH-sis*) Narrowing of the aortic valve, the valve between the lower left chamber of the heart, the left ventricle, and the large artery called the aorta. If this narrowing is severe, it places a significant burden on the heart.

AORTIC VALVE (*ay-OR-tik valv*) Valve preventing a leakage of blood back from the aorta into the left ventricle.

AORTOCORONARY SAPHENOUS VEIN BYPASS (*ay-OR-toh-KOR-oh-na-ree SAH-fe-nus*) *See* Coronary bypass.

ARRHYTHMIA (*ah-RITH-mee-ah*) Abnormal rhythm of the heartbeat, including fast, slow, and irregular rhythms and premature beats.

ARTERIAL BLOOD (*ar-TE-ree-al*) Blood carried in the arteries. The blood is bright red because it is rich in oxygen, which it receives in the lungs.

ARTERIOGRAMS (*ar-TE-ree-oh-grams*) *See* Coronary Arteriography, Angiocardiography, Angiogram, and Angiography.

ARTERIOLES (*ar-TE-ree-ols*) The smallest arterial blood vessels, resulting from repeated branching of the arteries, which carry blood from the arteries to the capillaries.

ARTERIOSCLEROSIS *(ar-TE-ree-oh-skle-ROH-sis)* Commonly called "hardening of the arteries." *See also* Atherosclerosis.

ARTERY *(AR-ter-ee)* Blood vessels that carry blood away from the heart to the various parts of the body.

ATHEROSCLEROSIS *(ATH-er-oh-skle-ROH-sis)* Narrowing within an artery, consisting of a yellowish material which contains cholesterol, fats, and other debris.

ATRIAL FIBRILLATION *(A-tree-al fi-bri-LA-shun)* Rhythm disturbance of the heart in which the atria no longer beat in their typical rhythmic fashion but rather quiver chaotically and ineffectively at extremely rapid rates. This produces an irregular and often rapid rhythm of the main pumping chambers of the heart, the ventricles.

ATRIUM *(A-tree-um)* One of the two upper receiving chambers of the heart, which collects the blood from the veins and then delivers it to the ventricles. Also termed auricle.

BLOOD Reddish fluid that flows through the veins and arteries of the body, carrying nutrients to the organs and tissues and carrying wastes to the liver, kidneys, and lungs. It is composed of a liquid called plasma and a series of particles, among which are the red cells that carry oxygen to the tissues, the white cells that fight infection in the body, and the platelets that are involved in the blood clotting process. *See also* Plasma.

BLOOD PRESSURE The pressure within the arteries. It is usually described by two numbers. The first is the *systolic pressure* produced when the left ventricle contracts and squeezes the blood out into the arterial system. The second is *diastolic pressure,* that which remains when the left ventricle is resting between beats. Hence, a pressure of 120/80 is read as "120 over 80," the first of the numbers being the systolic pressure and the second being the diastolic pressure.

BLOOD VESSELS The blood vessels consist of three types of branching hollow tubes. The *arteries* carry blood from the heart, branching into smaller and smaller sizes until they become arterioles and then *capillaries,* tiny vessels so small that they can be seen only with a microscope and that form a massive network, delivering the blood to all the cells of the body. After the tissues have received the blood, taking up its oxygen and food and giving up waste products, the blood returns via the *veins,* vessels that have much thinner walls than arteries and that, having collected the blood from all the body, deliver it back into the atria of the heart.

BRADYCARDIA *(brad-ee-KAR-dee-ah)* Abnormally slow heart rate. Generally less than sixty beats per minute.

CAPILLARIES *(KAP-i-lar-eez)* Extremely small blood vessels that form networks between arterioles and veins. It is through these vessels that the oxygen and nutrition carried by the blood diffuse to the tissues and organs of the body. *See* Blood vessels.

CARDIAC *(KAR-dee-ak)* Pertaining to the heart.

CARDIAC OUTPUT Amount of blood pumped by the heart in a one-minute period.

CARDIOLOGIST *(kar-dee-OL-oh-jist)* Physician specially trained to diagnose and treat heart disease.

CARDIOPULMONARY BYPASS *(KAR-dee-oh-PUL-moh-ner-ee)* Complex apparatus used during open-heart operations. This machine is connected to the heart and blood vessels and functions both as a pump and as a means of bringing oxygen to the blood, during the time the heart is being operated on, and is either partially or completely nonfunctioning.

CARDIOVASCULAR *(KAR-dee-oh-VAS-ku-lar)* Pertaining to the heart and blood vessels.

CARDIOVERSION *(KAR-dee-oh-VER-shun)* Correction of a rapid or irregular rhythm disturbance by the application of an electrical shock delivered to the heart through the chest wall.

CATHETER *(KATH-e-ter)* Thin tube inserted into a vein or an artery, usually in the arm or groin, and guided into the chambers of the heart. It is used to take samples of blood, to measure pressures within the heart chambers, and to inject angiographic dye.

CEREBROVASCULAR *(SER-ee-bro-VAS-ku-lar)* Pertaining to the blood vessels in the brain.

CHOLESTEROL *(koh-LES-ter-ol)* Fatlike substance found in many foods, especially meats, shrimp, and egg yolks; it is also manufactured by the body.

CHRONIC *(KRON-ik)* Used in the field of medicine to describe a disorder present for a prolonged period of time.

CIRCULATION *(ser-ku-LAY-shun)* The course of the blood throughout the body, in effect moving in a circle, from the heart, to the tissues, and then back to the heart.

CIRCULATORY *(SER-ku-lah-to-ree)* Pertaining to the heart, the blood vessels, and the circulation of the blood.

CIRCUMFLEX CORONARY ARTERY One of the three major coronary arteries. It feeds the left side and part of the back of the heart.

COAGULATION *(koh-ag-u-LAY-shun)* Process whereby blood changes from a liquid to a thickened or solid state, as in the formation of a blood clot.

COLLATERAL VESSELS (CORONARY) *(koh-LAT-er-al)* When a coronary artery becomes occluded and can no longer supply an adequate amount of blood to a portion of the heart, the remaining arteries may develop new branches to provide blood to the deficient area. These new branches are termed collateral vessels.

CONSTRICTION *(kon-STRIK-shun)* The narrowing of the inside diameter of a blood vessel.

CONGESTIVE HEART FAILURE *(kon-JES-tiv)* *See* Heart failure.

CORONARY *(KORE-oh-na-ree)* "A coronary" is another term given for a heart attack. The word technically refers to the heart.

CORONARY ANGIOGRAPHY *See* Angiocardiography and Coronary arteriography.

CORONARY ARTERIES Arteries that conduct blood to the heart muscle. There are three major coronary arteries. The *right* wraps around the right side of the heart to supply its back side. The *left anterior descending* crosses over the front of the heart. The *circumflex* goes around the left side of the heart. The circumflex and anterior descending branch off from the *left main coronary artery.*

CORONARY ARTERIOGRAM *(KORE-oh-na-ree ar-TE-ree-oh-gram)* The film or x-ray moving picture that is obtained by coronary arteriography.

CORONARY ARTERIOGRAPHY *(KORE-oh-na-ree ar-te-ree-OG-rah-fee)* Procedure whereby a special dye is injected into the coronary arteries so that x-ray moving pictures can be taken of the inside walls of these vessels to determine the presence, severity, and location of coronary artery narrowing or occlusion. The procedure is done by threading a small tube through an artery from the groin or arm to a location just above the heart. Dye is also injected into the left ventricle, in an effort to determine whether there has been any temporary or permanent damage to the pumping function of that chamber. *See also* Angiocardiography.

CORONARY BYPASS SURGERY Operation in which a bypass or detour is placed around one or more obstructed coronary arteries, usually by taking a vein (saphenous vein) from the aorta and grafting it to an area of the coronary artery beyond the obstruction, thus permitting a greater supply of blood to the heart.

CORONARY CARE UNIT Area of specialized intensive care in a hospital where patients with suspected or proven heart attacks are initially treated.

CORONARY OCCLUSION (*KORE-oh-na-ree ok-KLU-shun*) Obstruction in one of the branches of the coronary arteries which stops or slows down the flow of blood to some part of the heart muscle.

CORONARY THROMBOSIS (*KORE-oh-na-ree throm-BOH-sis*) Formation of a blood clot in a branch of one of the arteries which conducts blood to the heart muscle. It is a form of coronary occlusion that may lead to a heart attack.

COR-PULMONALE (*kore-pul-mo-NAL-ee*) Heart disease resulting from a disease of the lungs or of the blood vessels in the lungs.

CYANOSIS (*sigh-ah-NO-sis*) Blueness of the skin caused by insufficient amount of oxygen in the blood.

DEFIBRILLATOR (*dee-FI-bre-la-tor*) Machine that delivers an electrical shock to the patient's chest, with the objective of restoring the normal heart rhythm when there has been a rhythm disturbance.

DIABETES (*dye-ah-BEE-teez*) Also called *diabetes mellitus*. Disease in which the body is unable to use sugar normally, owing to insufficient amounts of a substance called insulin, normally produced by the pancreas. Diabetes may lead to coronary artery disease and heart attack.

DIASTOLE (*dye-AS-toh-lee*) Period of the heart cycle when the ventricles are not contracting but rather are resting between beats, filling up with the blood received by the atria.

DIETICIAN *(dye-e-TISH-an)*   Person skilled in the scientific use of diet in health and disease.

DILATATION *(dil-a-TAY-shun)*   Stretching, distension, or enlargement of the heart or blood vessels.

DIURESIS *(dye-u-REE-sis)*   Increased outflow of urine.

DIURETIC *(dye-u-RET-ik)*   Medication given to increase the amount of urine, utilized to remove excess salt and water from the body.

DYSPNEA *(DISP-nee-ah)*   Difficult or labored breathing, shortness of breath.

ECG   *See* Electrocardiogram.

EDEMA *(e-DEE-mah)*   Swelling, usually of the legs, occasionally of the arms or face, caused by presence of abnormally large amounts of fluid in the tissues of the body.

EKG   *See* Electrocardiogram.

ELECTROCARDIOGRAM *(e-LEK-troh-KAR-dee-oh-gram)*   Graphic record produced by the electrical voltage changes generated by the heart as it contracts and relaxes. Also called ECG or EKG.

ELECTROCARDIOGRAPH *(e-LEK-troh-KAR-dee-oh-graf)*   Instrument that records the electrical changes produced by the heart.

EMBOLUS *(EM-boh-lus)*   Blood clot or other substance that dislodges from the heart or a blood vessel and travels to and obstructs an artery located downstream. This event is termed an *embolism*.

ENDOCARDITIS *(en-doh-kar-DYE-tis)*   Infection of the heart valves.

EXERCISE TEST   Test of the heart's capacity to function and capacity of the coronary arteries to deliver a sufficient supply of blood to the heart during the work of exercise. This test is usually performed using a motor-driven treadmill or stationary bicycle, and changes in blood pressure, heart rate, and electrocardiogram are recorded. Abnormalities of one of these frequently develop when narrowing of the coronary arteries prevents an adequate supply of blood to the heart during exercise, a period when the needs of the heart are at their greatest.

EXTRASYSTOLE *(eks-trah-SIS-toh-lee)*   A contraction of the heart that occurs prematurely and interrupts briefly the normal rhythm of the heart. Also termed premature beats or ectopic beats.

FIBRILLATION *(fi-bri-LAY-shun)* Ventricular fibrillation is one type of cardiac arrest or stopping of the heart, where the ventricles no longer beat but rather quiver in an ineffective manner. The pumping action of the heart is therefore lost. *See* Atrial fibrillation.

FLUOROSCOPE *(FLOO-roh-skope)* X-ray instrument with which the physician can view the silhouette of the patient's organs and body structures that lie deep in the body.

HDL High-density lipoprotein. A substance that carries cholesterol in the blood and is capable of removing cholesterol from within a fatty plaque. Higher levels of HDL in the blood are protective against coronary disease.

HEART Muscular hollow organ in the chest containing four chambers; the principal pump of the body.

HEART BLOCK Interference in the transmission of electrical impulses within the heart, which can then result in irregular rhythms and slowing of the heartbeat.

HEART FAILURE Also called *congestive heart failure*. A condition whereby the pumping action of the heart is impaired, so that blood backs up into the lungs or other parts of the body. In addition, there is an inadequate delivery of blood and the nutrition that it carries to the tissues of the body.

HEART-LUNG MACHINE Machine through which the body's blood may be detoured in order to dispose of wastes and to acquire oxygen while the heart is opened for surgery. *See* Cardiopulmonary bypass.

HEMIPLEGIA *(hem-ee-PLEE-jee-ah)* Paralysis of one side of the body caused by damage to the opposite side of the brain.

HEMOGLOBIN *(HE-moh-gloh-bin)* Oxygen-carrying red pigment contained in the red blood cells.

HEMORRHAGE *(HEM-or-ij)* Loss of blood from a blood vessel. In internal hemorrhage, the blood passes into the tissues surrounding the ruptured blood vessel. In external hemorrhage, as in a cut on the skin, it is a bleeding to the outside of the body.

HYPERTENSION *(high-per-TEN-shun)* Commonly called "high blood pressure." An elevation of blood pressure above normal ranges (above 150/90).

HYPERCHOLESTEROLEMIA *(high-per-koh-LES-ter-ole-me-ah)* Elevation in the amount of cholesterol present in the blood.

HYPOTENSION *(high-poh-TEN-shun)* Low blood pressure; blood pressure below the normal range.

INFARCT *(IN-farkt)* Area of tissue that is damaged or dies as a result of having received an insufficient supply of blood. Frequently used in the phrase "myocardial infarct," referring to an area of the heart muscle that is damaged because of an insufficient flow of blood through the coronary arteries that normally had supplied it.

INTERNAL MAMMARY ARTERY An artery located under the breastbone, one end of which may be attached directly to the coronary artery during coronary bypass surgery.

ISCHEMIA *(is-KEE-mee-ah)* A local, usually temporary, lack of blood supply to some part of the body. Often it is caused by a constriction or an obstruction in the blood vessels supplying that area.

LDL Low-density lipoprotein. A substance that carries cholesterol in the bloodstream. High blood levels of LDL cholesterol increase the risk of cardiovascular disease.

LEFT MAIN CORONARY ARTERY Important coronary artery, originating from the aorta, which divides into two other major coronary arteries, the left anterior descending and circumflex coronary arteries.

LEFT VENTRICLE Main pumping chamber of the heart.

LIPID *(LIP-id)* Fat or fatlike substance. Two of the major lipids implicated in the cause of coronary artery disease are cholesterol and (perhaps less importantly) triglycerides. *See* Cholesterol, Triglycerides.

MALIGNANT HYPERTENSION *(mah-LIG-nant high-per-TEN-shun)* Very severe high blood pressure, causing rapid damage to the kidneys, heart, brain, and other organs.

MITRAL VALVE *(MYE-tral)* Valve preventing backflow from the left ventricle to the left atrium.

MURMUR Swishing or blowing sound in the heart, which usually is heard with the aid of a stethoscope and which may be either a normal finding or indicate some type of heart or valve disorder.

MYOCARDIAL INFARCTION *(mye-oh-KAR-dee-al in-FARK-shun)* Damaging of an area of the heart muscle, resulting from a reduction in the supply of blood reaching that area.

PACEMAKER *(PACE-make-er)*   Small mass of specialized cells located in the upper right chamber of the heart that creates the electrical impulses that cause the heart muscle to contract in a normal rhythmic fashion. The *artificial* electrical cardiac pacemaker is a device used to substitute for the heart's natural pacemaker, to speed the heartbeat by a series of rhythmic electrical impulses when the heart's own rhythm beats too slowly, as in the instance of heart block.

PALPITATION *(pal-pi-TAY-shun)*   Sensation of a fluttering, racing, or skipping of the heart noted by the patient.

PERICARDITIS *(per-i-kar-DYE-tis)*   Inflammation or irritation of the pericardium. Pericarditis may have many causes, one being a myocardial infarction.

PERICARDIUM *(per-i-KAR-dee-um)*   Thin sac that surrounds the heart.

PHLEBITIS *(fle-BYE-tis)*   Also called *thrombophlebitis*. Inflammation of a vein, usually in a leg. Sometimes a blood clot forms in the inflamed vein and subsequently is carried to a lung, where it becomes an obstruction termed a pulmonary embolus.

PLASMA *(PLAZ-mah)*   Liquid part of the blood left when the other elements, the red and white blood cells, are removed.

POLYUNSATURATED FAT   *(pol-ee-un-SAT-u-rat-ed)*   Fats that are usually liquid oils of vegetable origin. A diet with a high polyunsaturated-fat content tends to lower the amount of cholesterol in the blood slightly.

PREMATURE BEATS   *See* Extrasystole.

PROPHYLAXIS *(proh-fi-LAK-sis)*   Some form of preventive treatment.

PULMONARY ARTERY *(PUL-moh-ner-ee)*   Large artery that carries blood, low in oxygen, from the right ventricle to the lungs.

PULMONARY EDEMA *(PUL-moh-ner-ee e-DEE-mah)*   When congestive heart failure is severe, the fluid within the left heart backs up into the lungs, seeping into the tiny air sacs in the lung, producing severe and oftentimes sudden shortness of breath.

PULMONARY VEINS   Four veins that carry oxygen-rich blood from the lungs into the left upper chamber of the heart, the left atrium.

PULSE *(puls)* Expansion of an artery that results from the pumping of blood by the heart, which may be felt with the fingers when they are placed over an artery.

REGURGITATION *(ree-gur-ji-TAY-shun)* Backward flow of blood through a defective valve in the heart.

REHABILITATION *(re-hah-bil-i-TAY-shun)* Return of a person disabled by disease or accident to the maximum attainable physical, mental, emotional, social, and economic usefulness.

RHEUMATIC HEART DISEASE *(roo-MAT-ik)* Damage done to the heart, particularly the heart valves, as the result of one or more attacks of rheumatic fever.

RIGHT CORONARY ARTERY One of three major coronary arteries. It passes across the right side of the heart, then to the back of the heart, where it provides its major blood supply.

RIGHT VENTRICLE The pumping chamber of the heart which sends blood into the lungs, so that the blood may take up oxygen.

SALVAGE Preserving or keeping alive areas of heart muscle that are endangered with or undergoing a myocardial infarction.

SAPHENOUS VEIN *(SAF-en-us)* A vein taken from the leg and attached from the aorta to the coronary artery in order to detour blood past an obstruction during coronary bypass surgery.

SATURATED FAT *(SAT-u-rate-ed)* Fats most often of animal origin, such as those contained in milk, butter, and meats, which are usually solid at room temperature. They may raise the blood cholesterol.

SERUM *(SIR-rum)* Liquid part of the blood remaining after it is clotted; the red cells, white cells, and platelets have therefore been removed.

SPHYGMOMANOMETER *(sfig-moh-mah-NOM-e-ter)* Instrument consisting of an arm cuff and a measuring device used to record the blood pressure.

STETHOSCOPE *(STETH-oh-skope)* Instrument that amplifies the sounds within the body, usually employed by doctors and nurses to listen to a patient's heart and lungs.

STRESS TEST *See* Exercise test.

STROKE Lack of blood supply to some part of the brain, producing a weakness or paralysis in one or more limbs or a defect in speech.

SYMPTOM (*SIMP-tum*) Description by a patient of his own medical problem.

SYNCOPE (*SIN-koh-pee*) Fainting.

SYSTOLE (*SIS-toh-lee*) Period when the heart muscle contracts.

TARGET HEART RATE Desired heart rate to be attained during an exercise conditioning program.

TACHYCARDIA (*tak-ee-KAR-dee-ah*) Abnormally fast heart rate. Generally, a rate of over 100 beats per minute.

THALLIUM (*THAL-ee-um*) A radioactive isotope which, when injected during some exercise tests, aids in detecting the location and severity of coronary blockage.

THERAPIST (*THER-ah-pist*) Person skilled in the treatment of disease or disability.

THROMBOPHLEBITIS *See* Phlebitis.

THROMBOSIS (*throm-BOH-sis*) Formation or presence of a blood clot inside a blood vessel or a cavity of the heart.

THROMBOLYSIS (*throm-boh-LYE-sis*) Dissolving a clot within a blood vessel.

THROMBUS (*THROM-bus*) Blood clot that forms inside of a blood vessel or in the cavity of the heart.

TREADMILL TEST *See* Exercise test.

TRIGLYCERIDE (*try-GLIS-er-ide*) One type of fat or lipid, present in the blood and body tissues. Triglycerides have been considered to be important in the development of coronary artery disease, although evidence for this is less sound than that for cholesterol.

VASODILATOR (*vas-oh-DYE-late-or*) Any substance or drug that causes the muscles of the arteries to relax, dilating or widening the hollow passageway within these tubular structures.

VASOPRESSOR (*vas-oh-PRES-or*) Any agent or drug that causes the muscles of the arteries to contract, constricting the arteries and often raising the blood pressure.

VEIN (*vane*) Blood vessel that carries blood from the various parts of the body back to the heart.

VENA CAVA *(VEE-nah KAY-vah)* One of two large veins returning blood from the upper and lower parts of the body to the right upper chamber of the heart, the right atrium.

VENOUS BLOOD *(VEE-nus)* Blood returning from the tissues, which has given up its oxygen and therefore is a more purplish or bluish color.

VENTRICLES *(VEN-tri-kels)* The major pumping chambers of the heart. *See* Left ventricle and Right ventricle.

Further Explorations

Common Cardiovascular Drugs: Detailed Notes

THIS APPENDIX describes details about the most commonly used cardiovascular drugs. If your doctor puts you on any medicines, be sure to check to see if they are discussed. If not, there is a blank *Personal Drug Information Sheet* on page 187. Ask your Doctor or nurse to fill it out for you.

The drugs discussed below, categorized according to how they work, are drugs that:

- Lower blood pressure.

- Remove excess water from the body.

- Resupply the body with necessary potassium

- Correct irregular heart rhythms.

- Increase the pumping action of the heart.

- Prevent and treat angina pectoris.

- Lower blood-fat content.

- Slow down clotting of the blood.

Drugs That Lower Blood Pressure (Antihypertensives)

GENERIC NAMES (TRADE NAMES):	Alphamethyldopa (Aldomet), Reserpine (Serpasil), Guanethidine (Ismelin), Clonidine (Catapres), Guanabenz (Wytensin)
Form:	Tablet
Administration:	Orally
Action and Uses:	Reduce blood pressure by indirectly relaxing the muscular walls of the blood vessels
Possible Side Effects:	Variable, but may include: Drowsiness Depression Dizziness or fainting (especially when one stands up suddenly) Fatigue Difficulty sleeping Nasal stuffiness Change in sexual potency
Special Instructions:	The sudden discontinuation of Catapres may produce a severe rise in blood pressure and is therefore to be avoided.
GENERIC NAMES (TRADE NAMES):	Hydralazine (Apresoline), Prazosin (Minipress), Minoxidil (Loniten)
Form:	Tablet
Administration:	Orally
Action and Uses:	Lower blood pressure by directly relaxing the blood vessels
Possible Side Effects:	Dizziness Fainting (especially when one stands up suddenly) Sensation of flushing of the skin Edema Increased hair growth and skin pigment (Minoxidil)

GENERIC NAMES **(TRADE NAMES):**	Captopril (Capoten), Enalapril (Vasotec)
Form:	Tablet
Administration:	Orally
Action and Uses:	1. Inhibits the manufacture of a chemical substance in the blood which causes the blood vessel walls to constrict and thus elevate the blood pressure. By interfering with the production of this substance, these drugs lower blood pressure. 2. By dropping the blood pressure, the workload of the heart falls, so that the heart can then pump with greater ease and strength.
Side Effects:	Excessive fall in blood pressure. Recommend medical supervision with first dose. Kidney dysfunction Fall in white blood cell count Rash and itching Change in taste Headache, dizziness High blood potassium. Should be checked by a blood test. Swelling of face and tongue, throat constriction. Check with a physician immediately if these occur.
GENERIC NAME:	*Diuretics.* These are discussed in detail on page 207.
Action and Uses:	Lower blood pressure by increasing the outflow of salt and water by the kidneys, which decreases the amount of fluid present in the bloodstream, decompresses the system, and lets pressure in the

blood vessels fall. Also relax the walls of the vessels and thereby reduce the blood pressure.

GENERIC NAME:

Beta Blocking Drugs. These are discussed in detail on page 216.

Action and Uses:

Lowers blood pressure in two principal ways:
1. The amount of blood ejected by the heart with each beat is reduced so that the blood pressure within the arteries falls.
2. Some of these relax the blood vessel wall.

GENERIC NAME:

"Combination drugs"

Form:

Numerous tablets contain drugs from two or three of the categories listed above.

Drugs that Remove Excess Water from the Body (Diuretics or "Water Pills")

GENERIC NAMES
(TRADE NAMES):

Thiazides and similar drugs
Chlorothiazide (Diuril), Hydrochlorothiazide (Hydrodiuril) (Esidrix)
Others: (Enduron), (Naqua), (Naturetin), (Renese), (Zaroxolyn), Chlothalidone (Hygroton, Thalidone), Furosemide (Lasix), Ethacrinic Acid (Edecrin), Bumetanide (Bumex), Triamterene (Dyrenium), Spironolactone (Aldactone), Amiloride (Moduretic, Midador) (Dyazide) and Maxzide) contain combinations of two of the above drugs.

Form:	Tablet
Administration:	Orally
Action and Uses:	Remove excess amounts of water and salt from the body by causing increases in the amount of urination. Often used for this purpose in congestive heart failure. Also used to lower blood pressure of some patients.
Possible Side Effects:	1. Loss of the mineral potassium from the body can occur with most diuretics, but seldom with Dyazide, Dyrenium, Aldactone, Aldactazide, Maxzide, or Amiloride. Your physician may order a blood test to check your potassium from time to time, since a low potassium level may make your heart more irritable. 2. Muscle cramps Muscle weakness Loss of appetite Symptoms of gout
Special Instructions:	1. One of the liquid potassium preparations or foods rich in potassium are often used in conjunction with some of the diuretics to prevent the excessive loss of potassium from the body. This is especially important when one of the digitalis preparations also is being taken. 2. It is a good idea to weigh yourself daily, in the morning, to check the amount of water loss.

Drugs That Resupply the Body with Necessary Potassium

GENERIC NAME (TRADE NAMES):	Potassium (Potassium Chloride), (K-Lyte), (Slow-K), (Kato), (K-Lor), (Kay-Ciel), (Kaon), (Micro-K), (Klotrix)
Form:	Either a liquid or controlled-release tablet. Also comes as a powder that can be dissolved in water or juice.
Administration:	Orally
Action and Uses:	Resupply the body with the potassium it may have lost as the result of the action of a diuretic.
Possible Side Effects:	Gastrointestinal distress including nausea, vomiting, or diarrhea Loss of appetite Abdominal burning
Special Instructions:	1. Potassium is also found in many foods: oranges, melon, dried fruit, potatoes, pineapple, tomatoes, grapefruit, prunes, bananas, apricots, cabbage, raisins, cantaloupe, meats, poultry, or fish. These can be used as supplemental sources of potassium. 2. The medication often tastes bad and causes stomach upset. Taking it with fruit juice or changing brands of potassium may be helpful.

Drugs That Correct Irregular Heart Rhythms (Antiarrhythmics)

Special Instructions:	Rather than correct the problem, antiarrhythmic drugs occasionally can make rhythm abnormalities worse. If you note an increase in palpitations, rapid heart rate, or fainting spells with any of these drugs, contact your physician immediately.
GENERIC NAME (TRADE NAMES):	Quinidine (Quinaglute), (Cardioquin), (Duraquin)
Form:	Tablet
Administration:	Orally
Action and Uses:	Correct irregular heart rhythm, premature beats, and some types of very rapid heart action (tachycardias)
Possible Side Effects:	Gastrointestinal discomfort, including nausea, vomiting, or diarrhea Loss of appetite Ringing in ears Bruising (contact your physician)
GENERIC NAME (TRADE NAMES):	Procainamide (Pronestyl), (Procan-SR)
Form:	Capsule
Administration:	Orally
Action and Uses:	Correct irregular heart rhythm, premature beats, and some types of very fast heart rates (some tachycardias)
Possible Side Effects:	Gastrointestinal distress, including nausea, vomiting, or diarrhea Fever

Skin rash
Aching joints
Dizziness

Special Instructions:	Check with your doctor if you develop arthritis or aching joints.
GENERIC NAME (TRADE NAME):	Disopyramide (Norpace)
Form:	Capsule
Administration:	Orally
Action and Uses:	To correct irregular heart rhythm, premature beats, and some types of very fast heart rates (some tachycardias)
Possible Side Effects:	Dry mouth Constipation Difficulty with urination Dryness of eyes, nose and throat Loss of appetite Gas bloating Nervousness Fatigue Edema or weight gain
GENERIC NAME:	*Beta Blocking Drugs.* These are discussed in detail on page 216.
Form:	Tablet
Administration:	Orally
Action and Uses:	Slows the heart. Prevents and treats fast or irregular heartbeats, lowers blood pressure, prevents pain of angina pectoris.
GENERIC NAME (TRADE NAME):	Tocainide (Tonocard)
Form:	Tablet
Administration:	Orally
Action and Uses:	To correct irregular and rapid heart rhythms and premature beats

Possible Side Effects:	Dizzyness, giddiness, or tremulousness
	Disorientation or altered mood
	Uncoordination
	Gastrointestinal distress
	Rash
	Sweating

GENERIC NAME (TRADE NAME):	Mexilitine (Mexitil)
Form:	Capsule
Administration:	Orally
Action and Uses:	To correct irregular heart rhythms, premature beats and some types of very fast heart rhythms (tachycardias).
Possible Side Effects:	Tremor, dizziness, and uncoordination
	Change in sleep habits
	Headache
	Gastrointestinal upset
	Blurred vision or sun sensitivity
	Rash

GENERIC NAMES (TRADE NAMES):	Flecainide (Tambocor), Encainide
Form:	Tablet
Action and Uses:	To correct irregular or rapid heart rhythm and premature beats
Possible Side Effects:	Dizziness, headache, uncoordination
	Fatigue
	Visual Disturbances
	Gastrointestinal upset
	Shortness of breath
	Tingling of arms or legs

GENERIC NAME (TRADE NAME):	Amiodarone (Cordarone)

Form:	Tablet
Administration:	Orally
Action and Uses:	To correct irregular or rapid heart rhythm and premature beats.
Possible Side Effects:	Rash or pigmentation of the skin Gastrointestinal disturbances Deposits of material in the eye (check with an eye doctor) Changes in the function of the thyroid gland (*check with your doctor*) Shaking, dizziness, uncoordination Headache Scarring of the lung with shortness of breath
GENERIC NAMES:	*Calcium Channel Blocking Drugs.* These are discussed in detail on page 218.

Drugs That Increase Pumping Action of the Heart

GENERIC NAMES (TRADE NAMES):	Digitalis, Digoxin, Digitoxin (Lanoxin)
Form:	Tablet
Administration:	Orally
Action and Uses:	Increase the pumping strength of the heart in cases of congestive heart failure. Also, correct some forms of irregular or rapid heartbeats.
Possible Side Effects:	Gastrointestinal distress, including nausea, vomiting, or diarrhea Visual disturbances

Heart palpitations
Skipped or premature beats
Slowing of heart rate

Special Instructions:

1. If any of the above symptoms occur or if your heart rate drops below 50 beats per minute, *contact your physician*.

2. If you are taking water pills (diuretics), you may have an increased sensitivity to some of these side effects. If you are taking a digitalis preparation and a diuretic, your physician may have you take potassium to help avoid these side effects.

Drugs That Reduce the Workload of the Heart and Therefore Its Pumping Action

GENERIC NAMES
(TRADE NAMES):

Captopril (Capoten), Enalapril (Vasotec), Hydralazine (Apresoline), Prazosin (Minipress), Minoxidil (Loniten), See page 204 for information about these drugs.

Long-Acting Nitrates See page 216.

Nifedipine and other new calcium channel blocking drugs. See page 218.

Action and Uses:

These drugs relax the blood vessel walls causing blood pressure to fall and thus making it easier for the heart to pump. Because of the decrease in workload, these drugs reduce the size of an enlarged heart.

Drugs That Help Prevent and Treat Angina Pectoris (Antianginals)

GENERIC NAMES (TRADE NAMES):	*Short-Acting Nitrates:* Nitroglycerin (NTG), Glycerine trinitrate (NTG, Nitrostat, Nitrolinqual Spray)
Form:	Tablet or Spray
Administration:	Held under tongue or sprayed into mouth
Action and Uses:	To treat or prevent angina pain.
Possible Side Effects:	Headache or fullness in the head Flushing of the skin Dizziness and fainting (especially upon standing suddenly)
Special Instructions:	Nitroglycerin tablets must be kept in a well-sealed dark container supplied by your pharmacist or they will lose their potency in about 6 months.
GENERIC NAME (TRADE NAMES):	*Long-Acting Nitrates*
Form:	Tablet (Isordil, Dilatrate, Nitro-Bid Sorbitrate, Cardilate, Nitrospan) Ointment (Nitrol Ointment, Nitro-Stat Ointment) Patch (Nitro-Disc, Transderm Nitro, Nitro-Dur)
Administration:	Tablets are swallowed or held under the tongue. Ointment is rubbed onto skin and covered with a plastic wrap or tape. Patches are stuck onto the skin.
Action and Uses:	These drugs are not used for an acute angina attack as is sublingual (under the tongue) nitroglycerin, but used to *prevent* angina.

GENERIC NAMES (TRADE NAMES):	*Beta Blocking Drugs.* Propranolol (Inderal), (Inderal-LA), Atenolol (Tenormin), Nadolol (Corgard), Metoprolol (Lopressor), Timolol (Blocadren), Labetalol (Trandate) (Normodyne), Acebutolol (Sectral), Pindolol (Viskin)

Form: Tablet

Administration: Orally

Action and Uses: Prevents angina by decreasing the work of the heart — by slowing the heart rate, lowering the blood pressure, and relaxing the vigor of contraction of the heart. Slightly decreased risk of heart attack and cardiovascular mortality if taken after a myocardial infarction.

Possible Side Effects:
Gastrointestinal distress including nausea, vomiting, or diarrhea
Fatigue, sleepiness, difficulty sleeping, mental slowing
Shortness of breath
Wheezing
Slowing of heart rate to less than 50 beats per minute
Increase in body weight owing to retention of body fluids

Special Instructions: Your physician should be advised if you have shortness of breath, gain more than 4 pounds in a few days or detect an undue slowing of your heart rate. Some patients who have asthma or diabetes may have other side effects that can be discussed with a physician. This medication should not be stopped abruptly without advice from a physician if you have severe angina pain.

GENERIC NAMES (TRADE NAMES):	*Calcium Blocking Drugs* (Also called *calcium channel blocking drugs* or *calcium antagonists*) Nifedipine (Procardia, Adalat), Diltiazem (Cardizem), Verapamil (Calan, Isoptin)
Form:	Tablets and capsules
Administration:	Orally
Action and Uses:	1. Lowers the work of the heart by relaxing blood vessels, lowering blood pressure, slowing the heart rate and decreasing the force of the heart beat.
	2. Relieves coronary spasm.
	3. Improves certain rapid rhythm disturbances of the heart.
Possible Side Effects:	Dizziness, fainting, falling blood pressure
	Edema
	Nervousness, sleep changes
	Headache
	Slowing of the heart with Verapamil and Diltiazem
	Shortness of breath (mainly with Verapamil)
	Constipation
	Gastrointestinal upset

Drugs That Help Lower Blood-Fat Levels (Lipid-Lowering Drugs)

GENERIC NAMES (TRADE NAMES):	Cholestyranine (Questran), Colestipol (Colestid)
Form:	Powder
Administration:	Orally, dissolved in juice, beverage, applesauce, and so on.

Action and Uses:	Lowers the blood cholesterol
Possible Side Effects:	Constipation Abdominal discomfort Nausea Deficiencies in certain vitamins may occur (vitamins A, D, K), which may lead to bleeding tendencies. These are avoided by taking vitamin supplements under your physician's supervision.
Special Instructions:	Always mix with a liquid or semiliquid food. Use in conjunction with a low-cholesterol, low-fat diet. This drug may interfere with the actions of other medications, so that you should always check with your physician when taking other drugs.
GENERIC NAME **(TRADE NAME):**	Probucol (Lorelco)
Form:	Tablet
Administration:	Orally
Action and Use:	Lowers blood cholesterol
Possible Side Effects:	Gastrointestinal upset Dizziness and fainting Headache Rash Tingling of hands and feet
Special Instructions:	Oftentimes not used immediately after a heart attack
GENERIC NAME:	Niacin, Nicotinic Acid
Form:	Tablet or capsule
Administration:	Orally
Action and Uses:	Lowers blood cholesterol and triglycerides.
Possible Side Effects:	Flushing of the skin Itching

Gastrointestinal upset
Increased blood sugar

GENERIC NAME (TRADE NAME):	Gemfibrozil (Lopid)
Form:	Capsule
Administration:	Orally
Action and Uses:	Lowers blood triglycerides and may lower cholesterol slightly.
Possible Side Effects:	Gastrointestinal upset Rash Headache Dizziness Muscle aches
GENERIC NAME (TRADE NAME):	Clofibrate (Atromid-S)
Form:	Capsule
Administration:	Orally
Actions and Uses:	Lowers high levels of triglycerides and, in some cases, lowers high levels of cholesterol
Possible Side Effects:	Gallstones Nausea Loss of appetite Aching muscles Atromid-S may add to the effect of anticoagulants such as Coumadin, increasing the risk of bleeding Possible increased incidence of malignancy.

Drugs That Slow Down Clotting of Blood (Anticoagulants)

GENERIC NAMES (TRADE NAMES):	Warfarin, Dicumarol (Coumadin)
Form:	Tablet

Administration:	Orally
Action and Uses:	Slows down the clotting action in the blood to prevent the development of a blood clot or thrombus in an artery or a vein.
Possible Side Effects:	Bleeding: red urine, red or black bowel movement, excessive bleeding when cut, nose bleeds, bleeding gums Appearance of black and blue marks on the skin
Special Instructions:	If any of the above symptoms occur, contact your physician. A blood test called prothrombin time or Pro-time must be taken periodically to ensure that the correct amount of the drug is being taken. Many drugs such as aspirin, arthritis medications, sleeping pills, and antibiotics may interact with this drug, changing its potency and its effect. Check with your physician before taking any other medications.

Drugs That May Lessen Seriousness of a New Heart Attack

Can any medication lessen the seriousness of another heart attack, should one come along? There have been several clinical studies suggesting the possibility that one or another drug might just have such a desirable effect.

Drugs looked at by medical scientists include beta blockers, sulfinpyrazone (Anturane), dipyridamole (Persantine), and aspirin. Whether, when, and how much these drugs in fact work to lessen the likelihood of another heart attack occurring, or reduce its severity is still undecided, nor are we sure how these drugs would work. All but the beta blockers have the capacity of acting as a lubricant, making the blood less "sticky," less likely to thrombose, and because of the lubricating action, they are used after angioplasty and bypass surgery. Beta blocking drugs may prevent serious rhythm disturbances from occurring.

If you have been put on one of these drugs, fine. If not, that's O.K., too, since many physicians hesitate to use a medication until its benefits become clearly known.

Personal Drug Information Sheet

Ask your physician or nurse to fill this out for any drugs prescribed for you that are not discussed in this appendix.

Drug No. 1

SCIENTIFIC NAME:

TRADE NAME:

Form:

Administration:

Action and Uses:

Special Instructions:

Drug No. 2

SCIENTIFIC NAME:

TRADE NAME:

Form:

Administration:

Action and Uses:

Special Instructions:

Four Food Groups You Should Eat Every Day

THIS TABLE LISTS the four food groups that should be eaten most days in order to achieve a balanced diet. It shows the amount of food in each group necessary to provide a nutritious, balanced diet, providing all essential vitamins, minerals, proteins, carbohydrates, and necessary fats.

FOOD GROUP	CONTAINS	SUGGESTIONS FOR A SINGLE SERVING	SERVINGS PER DAY
1. Meat, poultry, fish, meat substitutes	Proteins, vitamins, minerals, fats, iron	4 oz. of fish, poultry, or lean meat. Substitutes: natural peanut butter, beans (kidney, lima, baked), split peas.	1 1
2. Vegetables and fruits	Vitamins, minerals, roughage	½ cup juice, 1 piece fruit, 1 cup vegetables	4
3. Breads and cereals	Proteins, vitamins, minerals, starches, bulk	1 slice bread, 1 cup flaked cereal, ½–⅔ cup cooked cereal	4
4. Dairy	Proteins, vitamins, minerals	1 glass nonfat milk, low-cholesterol cheese, cottage cheese, nonfat yogurt	2

Rearranging Your Menu

WHAT YOU USED TO EAT ON A TYPICAL DAY	WHAT YOU CAN EAT TODAY
Breakfast	
Orange juice	Orange juice
Cornflakes with fruit and milk	Cornflakes with fresh fruit and nonfat milk
Scrambled eggs	Scrambled low-cholesterol egg substitute
Sausage	Low-cholesterol sausage substitute
Toast and butter	Toast and corn-oil margarine (or a similar polyunsaturated margarine)
Milk	Nonfat milk
Coffee or tea with cream	Coffee or tea with nondairy creamer
Lunch	
Minestrone soup	Minestrone soup
Baked halibut with lemon	Baked halibut with lemon
Cottage cheese	Low-fat cottage cheese
Sliced zucchini	Sliced zucchini
Fresh fruit	Fresh fruit
Bread and butter	Bread and corn-oil margarine
Coffee or tea with cream	Coffee or tea with nondairy creamer

195

WHAT YOU USED TO EAT ON A TYPICAL DAY	WHAT YOU CAN EAT TODAY
Dinner	
Tomato juice	Tomato juice
Green salad with dressing	Green salad with low-fat dressing
Chicken	Roast chicken (skinned)
Mashed potatoes with butter	Mashed potatoes made with nonfat milk and corn-oil margarine
Green beans	Green beans
French bread and butter	French bread with corn-oil margarine
Pudding	Pudding made with nonfat milk
Ice Cream	Nonfat frozen yogurt
Wine, milk, or coffee	Wine, nonfat milk, or coffee

Shopping Suggestions:
How to Read Food Labels

ALL PACKAGED FOOD processors are required to identify the ingredients in their products. By using your knowledge of calories, fats, and cholesterol, you may select for use only those food products that will help provide good nutrition without risk. For example:

Black Forest Cake—Prepared and Ready-to-Bake

INGREDIENTS: Cherries, sugar, modified whey, corn syrup, enriched flour, fresh whole milk, fresh whole eggs, vegetable shortening, heavy whipping cream, Grade AA butter, chocolate, cocoa, mono- and diglycerides, baking powder, modified food starch, vegetable gum, vanilla, salt, gelatin, ascorbic acid, skim milk, lecithin, vegetable color.

COMMENT: *Caution*—note the milk, cream, eggs, shortening, butter, and chocolate.

Buttermilk Biscuits (Refrigerated)

INGREDIENTS: Enriched bleached flour, water, beef fat, dextrose, hydrogenated vegetable oil, baking soda, salt, corn starch, artificial flavoring.

COMMENT: *Caution*—watch the hydrogenated oil and beef fat.

Mayonnaise (Imitation)

INGREDIENTS: Water, soybean oil, vinegar, egg yolk, modified food starch, salt, mustard flour, spices, natural flavor.

COMMENT: *Caution*—contains egg yolks. Regular mayonnaise contains eggs but is acceptable when used in moderation because the amount of egg is small.

Minestrone Soup (Canned)

INGREDIENTS: Beef stock, carrots, potatoes, water, celery, beans, zucchini, salt, potato starch, hydrolyzed plant protein, cheddar cheese and natural flavoring.

COMMENT: The ingredients basically are good from the point of view of cholesterol and saturated fats, but canned soups are very salty.

Pancake Mix (Refrigerated)

INGREDIENTS: Skim milk, enriched flour, liquid sugar, pasteurized whole eggs, margarine, corn syrup, buttermilk solids, baking powder, salt, whey solids.

COMMENT: *Caution*—this batter contains eggs.

Peanut Butter

INGREDIENTS: Peanuts, dextrose, hardened vegetable oils, sugar.

COMMENT: *Caution* — the hardened vegetable oils are heavy in saturated fat content.

Peanut Butter, Natural

INGREDIENTS: Peanuts

COMMENT: This is O.K.

Pudding Mix (Powdered)

INGREDIENTS: Sugar, dextrose, cornstarch, modified cornstarch, salt, vegetable gum, artificial flavor, natural flavor, artificial color.

COMMENT: *Caution* — the content of sugar may be high, and this may be undesirable if you are overweight or have high triglycerides. Pudding made with whole milk is, of course, high in saturated fat. Instant puddings are very high in salt content.

Tomato Catsup

INGREDIENTS: Tomatoes, sugar, corn syrups, vinegar, salt, dehydrated onion, garlic, spices, and flavoring.

COMMENT: Looks good.

Of course, if you're on a low-salt diet, you should watch for this on the labels, too.

Dining Out

PEOPLE TEND to take extreme positions about the idea of eating out. Either they think it is nearly impossible (in the United States at least) to avoid loading up on cholesterol, saturated fats, and salt in a restaurant or else they think that if you *do* get a cholesterol-free meal, it will be as bland as the Child's Plate. Some people react by simply having the same rich meals when they eat out that they always have.

There is no need for that. Although the amount of cholesterol and saturated fats that you end up with in the fast-food hamburger franchises is often excessive, in most cases, whether you are in a diner or a five-star restaurant, it is rare that there is a lack of acceptable choice in selections—and certainly not in many of the restaurants with ethnic cuisines such as Oriental and Central and Latin American. Another point: remember that when you are eating out, you're often inclined to treat it as a festive celebration and gorge on food and drink. But of course you don't have to.

Here are some foods you can order when you're in a restaurant:

Appetizers and Snacks

Carrots

Celery

Crab cocktail

Oyster or shrimp cocktail

Fruit cup

Juice, vegetable or fruit

Mushrooms

Nuts

Pickled herring (avoid if on a low-salt diet)

Radishes

Salads (see below)

Salads

Dressings: Use oil and vinegar or any other not made with eggs, cream, or cheeses.

Cottage cheese salads

Fruit salads, all kinds

Vegetable salads, all kinds

Soups

Bean

Clam chowder, Coney Island (red kind, not Boston)

Consommé

Gazpacho, without sour cream

Onion

Pea

Avoid soups made with cream such as bisques. Avoid bouillon if you're following a low-salt diet.

Entrees

Entrees are best if broiled or roasted. Avoid rich sauces and gravies made with fat, cream, or butter.

Beef (choose the leanest cuts)

Chicken

Fish (not deep fried)

Lamb

Shellfish (crab, lobster, scallops, clams, oysters)

Turkey

Veal

Side Dishes

Mushrooms

Potatoes (including sweet potatoes and yams)

Rice

Spaghetti

Vegetables

These should not be made with butter or cream sauce.

Desserts

Angel Food cake

Baked apple

Melon and other fruit, canned, fresh, or frozen

Sherbets, sorbets

Yogurt, low-fat frozen

Jell-o

Beverages

Alcoholic beverages, beer, and wine (in moderation)

Buttermilk, low-fat

Carbonated beverages

Coffee

Fruit juices

Nonfat milk

Powdered cocoa with nonfat milk

Tea

Sandwiches

Bread should not be made from egg. Sandwich may contain margarine, mayonnaise, catsup, or mustard.

Chicken

Fish

Lettuce

Sprouts

Tomato

Tuna or tuna salad

Turkey

Breakfast Foods

Cereals should be served with nonfat milk.

Cooked cereals, such as oatmeal, Cream of Wheat, Cream of Rice

Dry cereals such as Puffed Rice, Shredded Wheat, Wheaties

Toast or muffin with margarine or jam

Caloric Content of Foods

FOOD	PORTION	CALORIES
Beverages, Alcoholic		
Beer	1 cup (8 oz.)	115
Brandy	1 oz.	70
Eggnog	½ cup	335
Highball	1 cup	165
Port, vermouth, muscatel	½ cup	155
Rum	1 jigger (1½ oz.)	140
Whiskey	1 jigger (1½ oz.)	130
Wine, white, rose	½ cup	85–105
Beverages, Nonalcoholic		
Carbonated soft drinks	1 cup (8 oz.)	80
Chocolate milk	1 cup	200
Cocoa	1 cup	175
Coffee, black	1 cup	1
with cream and sugar		
(1 teaspoon each)	1 cup	45
Tea	1 cup	1
Cereals, Cereal Products		
Bread		
Boston, enriched, brown	2 large slices	200
corn or muffins, enriched	2	220
raisin, enriched	2 slices	130
rye, American	2 slices	110

FOOD	PORTION	CALORIES
white, enriched	2 slices	120
whole-wheat	2 slices	110
Bread, rolls, sweet, unenriched	1	320
Cornflakes	1 cup	100
Crackers		
graham	2	60
saltines	2	30
soda	10 oyster	40
Macaroni, cooked	½ cup	70
Noodles, cooked	1 cup	100
Oatflakes, cooked	1 cup	75
Pancakes, wheat	2 cakes	150
Pie	1 slice	300–400
Popcorn, popped	1 cup	60
Pretzels	15 small sticks	15
Rice, cooked	½ cup	75
Spaghetti	1 cup cooked	220
Tapioca, cooked	½ cup	130
Waffles	1 waffle	225
Wheat germ	1 cup	365
Confectionary, Sugar		
Chocolate, sweetened	2½ oz. bar	335
milk	4 oz.	542
plain	4 oz.	471
Chocolate creames	2	110
Fudge	1 piece	120
Honey	1 tablespoon	65
Jams	1 tablespoon	55
Jellies	1 tablespoon	50
Jelly beans	10 pieces	70
Molasses	1 tablespoon	150
Syrup (chiefly corn syrup)	½ cup	427
Sugar, maple	1 tablespoon	55
cane or beet	1 tablespoon	50
Dairy Products, Eggs		
Cheese, cheddar	1″ square	115
cottage	½ cup	100
cream	2 tablespoons	100
limburger	2 tablespoons	100
parmesan	2 tablespoons	110
roquefort	2 tablespoons	105

FOOD	PORTION	CALORIES
Swiss	2 tablespoons	105
Cream, light	1 tablespoon	30
heavy, or whipping	1 tablespoon	50
Eggs, whole	1 medium	75
Egg white, raw	1 medium	15
Egg yolk, raw	1 medium	60
Milk, pasteurized, whole	1 cup	165
buttermilk, cultured	1 cup	80
canned, evaporated,	½ cup	140
unsweetened, condensed,	½ cup	480
sweetened, nonfat	1 cup	80
Goat's milk	½ cup	71
Ice cream	½ cup	150
Fats, Oils		
Butter	1 tablespoon	100
Mayonnaise	1 tablespoon	100
Olive oil	1 tablespoon	125
Peanut butter	1 tablespoon	85
All other oils	1 tablespoon	135
Fruit, Fruit Juices		
Apples	1 sweet	60–90
Apple juice, fresh	1 cup	120
Apple sauce, sweetened	½ cup	80
Apricot	1 medium	18
Avocados	1 fresh	370
Bananas	1 (about 6 in.)	94
Blackberries, fresh	½ cup	40
canned, sweetened	½ cup	85
Blueberries, fresh	½ cup	45
canned, sweetened	½ cup	110
Cantaloupe	½ fresh	40
Cherries, canned, sweetened	½ cup	100
Cranberry sauce	2 tablespoons	60
Dates, dried	5 pitted	100
Fruit cocktail, canned	½ cup	80
Grapes, fresh	½ cup	68
Grape juice	½ cup	75
Grapefruit	½ (4¼″ dia.)	75
Grapefruit juice, fresh	½ cup	45
Lemons	1 fresh, 2″	30
Olives, green	4 medium	40
Oranges, fresh	1 orange, 3″	70
Orange juice, fresh	½ cup	55

FOOD	PORTION	CALORIES
Peaches, fresh	1 medium, 2½″	45
canned, sweetened	2 halves	85
Pears	1 pear, 2½″	95
Pineapple, canned, sweetened	½ cup	100
Pineapple juice, canned	½ cup	60
Plums	1 plum, 2″	30
Prunes, dried, uncooked	4 large	110
Raisins, dried	½ cup	190
Raspberries, fresh	½ cup	50
canned, sweetened	1 cup	100
Strawberries, fresh	10 large	35
frozen, sweetened	½ cup	125
Meat, Poultry (raw unless otherwise stated)		
Bacon, medium fat, cooked	2 strips	100
Beef (medium fat)		
hamburger, cooked	¼ lb.	225
rib roast, cooked	2 slices (lean-fat)	200–400
rump, cooked	2 slices	190
sirloin, cooked	¼ lb. (lean-fat)	200–300
canned, corned	4 oz.	240
liver	1 slice	85
Chicken		
fried	¼ lb.	275
broiled	¼ lb.	218
liver	¼ lb.	85
Ham		
boiled	¼ lb.	300
smoked, cooked	¼ lb.	400
canned, spiced	¼ lb.	290
Lamb (medium fat)		
leg roast, cooked	¼ lb.	270
rib chop, cooked	¼ lb.	140
Pork (see also Bacon and Ham)		
medium fat	¼ lb.	365
loin or chops, cooked	1 chop	265
Turkey, medium fat	¼ lb.	270
Veal, medium fat	¼ lb. (cutlet-roast)	220–360
Venison	¼ lb.	140
Nuts		
Almonds, salted	15 nuts	100
Brazil nuts	5 nuts	100
Cashew nuts, roasted or cooked	10 nuts	200

FOOD	PORTION	CALORIES
Chestnuts	2 large nuts	30
Peanuts, roasted	½ cup	440
Pecans	1 tablespoon	52
Walnuts	2 tablespoons	95
Sea Food (raw unless otherwise stated)		
Clams, long and round	¼ lb.	80
Cod	1 piece	70
Crab, canned or cooked, meat only	½ cup	85
Flounder	¼ lb.	200
Frog legs	3 large	200
Haddock	¼ lb.	200
Halibut	¼ lb.	200
Lobster	1 (¾ lb.)	300
Oysters	5–8 medium	80
Salmon		
Pacific, cooked	¼ lb.	180
canned	½ cup	190
Sardines, canned in oil	5 medium	180
Scallops, fried	5–6 medium	425
Shrimps, canned, drained	10–12 medium	45
Trout	¼ lb. (brook-lake)	210–290
Soup		
Broth	1 cup	25
Bean	1 cup	260
Beef	1 cup	115
with vegetables	1 cup	80
Chicken noodle	1 cup	68
Lentil	1 cup	600
Pea, creamed	1 cup	270
Tomato	1 cup	100
Vegetable	1 cup	90
Vegetables		
Asparagus, canned	½ cup	25
Beans		
kidney	½ cup	90
lima, fresh	½ cup	90
canned	½ cup	95
snap, fresh	1 cup	35
wax, canned	½ cup	20
Beets (beetroots), peeled, fresh	½ cup	35
Broccoli, fresh	½ cup	20

FOOD	PORTION	CALORIES
Brussels sprouts, fresh	½ cup	30
Cabbage, fresh	wedge	25
Carrots, canned	½ cup	30
fresh	1 carrot, 6″	20
Cauliflower, fresh		25
Celery, stalk	2 stalks	17
Corn, fresh	1 ear (w/butter)	90
canned	½ cup	70
Cucumbers	½ cup, 7½″	20
Eggplant, fresh	½ cup	25
Kale, fresh	1 cup	40
Lentils	½ cup	110
Lettuce, headed, fresh	¼ head	15
Mushrooms (field mushrooms)	½ cup	20
Onions	1 onion, 2½″	40
Peas, green, fresh	½ cup	60
canned	½ cup	70
Peppers, green, fresh	1 large	24
Potato chips	7–10	110
Potatoes, raw	1 medium	90
dehydrated	½ cup	93
french fried	20 pieces	275
Radishes, fresh	4 small	10
Rhubarb, fresh	½ cup	10
Spinach, canned	½ cup	25
Sweet potatoes, fresh	1 small	150
candied	1 medium	300
canned	½ cup	120
Tomatoes	1 medium	35
canned	½ cup	25
Tomato catsup	2 tablespoons	40
Tomato juice, canned	½ cup	25
Miscellaneous		
Gelatin, dry, plain	1 tablespoon	35
dessert	½ cup	60
Yeast, compressed baker's	1 cake	10
Salad dressing		
(French-Thousand Island)	1 tablespoon	60–100

Source: B. J. Sharkey, *Physiological Fitness and Weight Control*, p. 118. Copyright 1974 by Mountain Press Publishing Co., Missoula, Mont. Reprinted by permission.

Calories Expended in Various Physical Activities

ACTIVITY	CAL/MIN
Standing, light activity	2.6
Washing and dressing	2.6
Washing and shaving	2.6
Driving a car	2.8
Washing clothes	3.1
Walking indoors	3.1
Shining shoes	3.2
Making bed	3.4
Dressing	3.4
Showering	3.4
Driving motorcycle	3.4
Metal working	3.5
House painting	3.5
Cleaning windows	3.7
Carpentry	3.8
Farming chores	3.8
Sweeping floors	3.9
Plastering walls	4.1
Truck and automobile repair	4.2
Ironing clothes	4.2

ACTIVITY	CAL/MIN
Farming, planting, hoeing, raking	4.7
Mixing cement	4.7
Mopping floors	4.9
Repaving roads	5.0
Gardening, weeding	5.6
Stacking lumber	5.8
Stone masonry	6.3
Pick-and-shovel work	6.7
Farming, haying, plowing with horse	6.7
Shoveling (miners)	6.8
Chopping wood	7.5
Gardening, digging	8.6
Walking upstairs	8–15
Pool or Billiards	1.8
Canoeing: 2.5 m.p.h.–4 m.p.h.	3.0–7.0
Volleyball: Recreational–Competitive	3.5–8.0
Golf: Foursome–Twosome	3.7–5.0
Horseshoes	3.8
Baseball (except pitcher)	4.7
Ping pong–Table tennis	4.9–7.0
Calisthenics	5.0
Rowing: Pleasure–Vigorous	5–15
Cycling: 5–15 m.p.h. (10 speed)	5–12
Skating: Recreation–Vigorous	5–15
Archery	5.2
Badminton: Recreational–Competitive	5.2–10
Basketball: Half–Full Court (more for fast break)	6–9
Bowling (while active)	7.0
Tennis: Recreational–Competitive	7–11
Water skiing	8.0
Soccer	9.0
Snowshoeing (2.5 m.p.h.)	9.0
Handball and squash	10.0
Mountain climbing	10.0
Judo and karate	13.0
Football (while active)	13.3
Wrestling	14.4
Skiing:	
Moderate to steep	8–12
Downhill racing	16.5
Cross-country: 3–8 m.p.h.	9–17

ACTIVITY	CAL/MIN
Swimming:	
Pleasure	6.0
Crawl: 25–50 yds/min.	6–12.5
Butterfly: 50 yds/min.	14.0
Backstroke: 25–50 yds/min.	6–12.5
Breaststroke: 25–50 yds/min.	6–12.5
Sidestroke: 40 yds/min.	11.0
Dancing:	
Modern: Moderate–Vigorous	4.2–5.7
Ballroom: Waltz–Rumba	5.7–7.0
Square	7.7
Walking	
Road–Field (3.5 m.p.h.)	5.6–7.0
Snow: Hard–Soft (3.5–2.5 m.p.h.)	10–20
Uphill: 5–10–15% (3.5 m.p.h.)	8–11–15
Downhill: 5–10% (2.5 m.p.h.)	3.6–3.5
15–20% (2.5 m.p.h.)	3.7–4.3
Hiking: 40 lb. pack (3.0 m.p.h.)	6.8
Running	
12 min. mile (5 m.p.h.)	10.0
8 min. mile (7.5 m.p.h.)	15.0
6 min. mile (10 m.p.h.)	20.0
5 min. mile (12 m.p.h.)	25.0

Source: B. J. Sharkey, *Physiological Fitness and Weight Control*, p. 128. Copyright 1974 by Mountain Press Publishing Co., Missoula, Mont. Reprinted by permission.

Energy Values for Various Physical Activities

THE ENERGY VALUES in these tables are expressed in terms of METs. 1 MET is equivalent to the energy consumed by the body when it is at rest.

ENERGY (METS)	BASIC ACTIVITY	WORK ACTIVITY	LEISURE ACTIVITY
1	Bed rest Sitting Talking Eating	Reading	Reading Watching TV Sewing
1–2	Brushing teeth Shaving Washing hands and face Dressing Strolling on level ground	Sweeping floors Ironing or making bed Washing dishes Typing Driving car	Driving auto Model building Walking
2–3	Walking on level ground, 2 m.p.h. Tub bathing	Light housekeeping Cooking Driving truck Using hand tools Auto repair Waxing floors	Fishing Walking on level ground Golf with power cart Boating

215

ENERGY (METS)	BASIC ACTIVITY	WORK ACTIVITY	LEISURE ACTIVITY
3–4	Shower bathing Brisk walking, 3 m.p.h. Sexual Intercourse	General house- keeping Farm work Assembly-line work Driving large truck	Golf with pull cart Brisk walking Slow bicycling, 6 m.p.h. Light gardening Horseback riding Sailing Bowling
4–5	Calisthenics Walking, 3.5 m.p.h.	Heavy housework Heavy gardening Lifting and carrying 30 lb. objects Home repairs	Tennis, doubles Heavy gardening Moderate bicycling Slow swimming Dancing Golf, carrying clubs
5–6	Quick walking, 4 m.p.h.	Sawing wood Working heavy tools Lifting and carrying 50 lb. objects Light shoveling Mowing lawn	Fast bicycling Ice skating Hiking Softball Square dancing Hunting
6–7	Jogging, 5 m.p.h.	Shoveling snow Chopping wood	Canoeing Tennis, singles Scuba diving Light downhill skiing Waterskiing
7–8	Climbing stairs Light jogging	Moving heavy objects Lifting and carrying 70 lb. objects	Skiing downhill Paddleboard Swimming backstroke Basketball Ice hockey Mountain climbing
8–9		Lifting and carrying 100 lb. objects	Running, 5½ m.p.h. Handball Swimming breast- stroke Cross-country skiing
10 and over			Fast running, 6 m.p.h. Gymnastics Football Snow sledding

Acknowledgments

WE ARE INDEBTED to a great many people for their constructive suggestions.

The following critiqued the original manuscript in its entirety: Hillel Abel, M.D.; Kanu Chatterjee, M.D.; Melvin Cheitlin, M.D.; Robert DeBusk, M.D.; Jack Edelen, M.D.; James F. Freis, M.D.; William Hancock, M.D.; William Haskell, Ph.D.; Gary Marcus, M.D.; Lani Moskowitz Strom, R.N.; Pate Thomson, M.D.; and Marianna Pieck, R.N.

Sections of this edition were reviewed by: Jill Caire, Ph.D.; Lawrence Duke, M.D.; Philip Frost, M.D.; W. McFate Smith, M.D.; Audrey Paulbitski, R.D.; Jill Schlesinger; Donna Silsbee, R.P.T.; Mindy Schwartz, R.N.; and Jane Tien, R.D.

And special thanks to Catherine and Suzanne Duke for being such quiet girls during the rewrite of this book.

We are also grateful to William Patrick at Addison-Wesley, for having the confidence to publish the second edition.

Finally, we want to express our greatest appreciation to Brian Williams for his help and expertise in editing and producing the book. His organizational and phrase-making abilities, we feel, enormously helped to improve the manuscript.

Index

Italic page numbers indicate illustrations. **Boldface** page numbers indicate glossary entries.